EXTENDED MATCHING QUESTIONS FOR THE MRCS

Cover Illustration by Michael D Robinson

DOGGER

EXTENDED MATCHING QUESTIONS FOR THE MRCS

Sunil Auplish
MBBS BSc (Hons)
Rickmansworth
Herts

M. K. Hossain-Ibrahim
MBBS BSc (Hons)
Russell Square
London

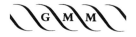

© 2001 Greenwich Medical Media

Greenwich Medical Media Ltd
137 Euston Road
London
NW1 2AA

ISBN 1 84110 062 5

First published 2001

A catalogue record for this book is available from the British Library.

Typeset by Phoenix Photosetting, Chatham, Kent

Visit our website at: www.greenwich-medical.co.uk

Printed by Alden Press

Contents

Preface   vii
Foreword   ix
Questions   x

Core Module 1:   Peri-operative Management 1   1

Core Module 2:   Peri-operative Management 2   23

Core Module 3:   Trauma   45

Core Module 4:   Intensive Care   67

Core Module 5:   Neoplasia   89

System Module A: Locomotor System   111

System Module B: Vascular   133

System Module C: Head, Neck, Endocrine and
                          Paediatric   155

System Module D: Abdomen   177

System Module E: Urinary System and Renal
                          Transplantation   203

Index   225

Preface

The new MRCS examination has introduced the extended matching question (EMQ), which many candidates may not be familiar with. We hope that this book gives you not only the chance to practice this type of question, but also will cover essential parts of the examination syllabus. Having so recently passed the examination we have based the questions not only on the format, but also on the questions that our peers and we could remember from recent examinations (with subtle changes).

The answer section includes information that is frequently tested, but which we often had difficulty in locating while revising. We hope that the tables and line diagrams will be a useful reference source during revision.

The book follows the STEP course closely with each chapter representing one of the ten modules. Although not everything could be covered here, we have endeavoured to include the topics felt as important and likely to be asked by the examiners.

EMQs aim to determine how well the candidate can **apply** their knowledge of surgery, rather than being a simple factual test. The Royal College of Surgeons suggests that one spends 45 min of the 2-h examination on the EMQ section, which equates to just over one-third of the examination. Each question has a theme printed at the top of the page, followed by a list of up to ten options from which to select the appropriate answer from the question printed below. You will be asked to choose **the single best** answer, whether this is a diagnosis, treatment plan or anatomical structure. In this manner, it is possible to test your clinical acumen and ability to prioritise.

This is the area of the examination where one can fall behind other candidates. With MCQs there is a 50% chance of getting the answer correct if you guess, whereas with EMQs this may be as low as 10%. However, even if you do not know the answer, it is usually possible to exclude many of the options and increase the likelihood of picking the right option.

The advice offered here about the examination is based on what was experienced by our peers and us.

- Do not run out of time – this is easier than you think, especially if the MCQ section is tricky and has taken more time than expected. The EMQ section is the last part of the paper and easy to forget about until you get to it.
- Look at **every** word – the questions have been carefully chosen and are carefully spelled out. A coal miner has different risk factors for disease than a publican.

- There is no negative marking so **answer every question!** If you are about to run out of time, fill in the answer sheet randomly – you may get a few marks.

We hope you find this book useful and wish you all the best in the forth-coming examinations.

K. H-I. and S. A.

Foreword

The extended matching question (EMQ) is a new style of examination for surgical candidates. Whether you like it or not, you have to face up to this format of examination and to conquer it if any progress is to be made in your career in surgery.

Much of the success in achieving the pass depends on a combination of common sense and clinical experience. If you have never encountered the clinical situation described in an EMQ, or indeed anything remotely like it, you are going to have to rely on what you can remember from your textbooks and from the STEP course text, which I sincerely hope you have studied carefully. So, it is important for you, in your examination preparation, to see as much clinical practice as is humanly possible. There is no substitute for it!

The possessors of this book are fortunate, because its authors, who I had the pleasure of teaching when they were anatomy demonstrators at Guy's Hospital in London, have collated a very useful collection of EMQs based on the MRCS examination, and, more importantly, discussed the answers in a clear and logical manner.

I answered most of the questions correctly when I read through the manuscript, but I also benefited a great deal from the useful comments after each question.

I commend this book to you all and wish you good luck in your exam.

Harold Ellis CBE, MCh, FRCS

Questions

Core Module 1
1. Pre-operative investigations
2. Problems with medication
3. Microbiology
4. Antibiotics
5. Use of local anaesthetic agents
6. Biopsy
7. Sterilisation and disinfection
8. Sutures
9. Wound infection
10. Complications of abdominal laparoscopic surgery

Core Module 2
1. Surgical dressings
2. Acid–base balance
3. Nutrition
4. Anaemia
5. Bleeding disorders
6. Postoperative shortness of breath
7. Postoperative pyrexia
8. Postoperative nerve palsies
9. Analgesia
10. Infection in the immunocompromised patient

Core Module 3
1. Diagnosis in primary survey
2. Hypovolaemic shock
3. Head injury
4. Glasgow Coma Score
5. Traumatic injury of the peripheral nervous system
6. Fracture management
7. Complications of fractures
8. Spinal injuries
9. Tendon anatomy and injury
10. Burns

Core Module 4
1. Chest conditions
2. Complications of central venous cannulation
3. Shock
4. Anatomy of the diaphragm

5. Lung volumes
6. Respiratory failure
7. Applied anatomy of the great vessels
8. Metabolic abnormalities
9. Ward allocation
10. Anatomy of the thorax

Core Module 5
1. Colorectal cancer
2. Tumour markers
3. Cytotoxic chemotherapy
4. Skin lesions
5. Breast lumps
6. Breast cancer
7. Oncogenes
8. Thyroid neoplasia
9. Lung cancer
10. Care of the terminally ill patient

System Module A
1. Around the wrist
2. Lower limb nerve injuries
3. Management of open fractures
4. The shoulder
5. Bone diseases
6. Fractures of the femur
7. Child with a limp
8. The knee
9. Brachial plexus injuries
10. Bone cysts and neoplasms

System Module B
1. Lower limb vascular disease
2. Lower limb amputation
3. Treatment of arterial occlusion
4. Anatomy of the lower limb
5. Aneurysms
6. Upper limb anatomy
7. Splenomegaly
8. Leg ulcers
9. Aortic aneurysms
10. Carotid endarterectomy

System Module C
1. Respiratory tract
2. Salivary glands
3. Sites of upper aerodigestive tract obstruction

4. Lumps in the neck
5. Complications of thyroid surgery
6. Epistaxis
7. Adrenal pathophysiology
8. Paediatric constipation
9. Abdominal conditions in children
10. Paediatric urogenital conditions

System Module D
1. Hernia anatomy
2. Abdominal incisions
3. Abdominal stomas
4. Dysphagia
5. Acute abdominal pain
6. Haematemesis
7. Abdominal masses
8. Mass in the right iliac fossa
9. Rectal bleeding
10. Hepatobiliary system

System Module E
1. Haematuria
2. Renal physiology
3. Management of renal tract calculi
4. Urological anatomy
5. Testicular conditions
6. Anatomy of the pelvis
7. Staging of bladder cancer
8. Renal function
9. Carcinoma of the prostate
10. Transplantation

Acknowledgements

For the preparation of this book, we are indebted to a number of people. Thanks must first be given to our tutors at Guy's Hospital Anatomy Department: Professor Harold Ellis and Mr Roger Parker, as well as the staff of the Dissection Room and the Gordon Museum at Guy's for their aid and patience. Too many colleagues to mention helped with ideas, and though not individually mentioned, your thoughts were most certainly needed. Thanks also to the unique artistry of Mike Robinson for the front cover illustration.

Finally, the book would not be here for everyone to enjoy were it not for both of our families, whom we thank for their guidance, enthusiasm and encouragement.

K. H-I & S.A.

Core Module 1: Peri-operative Management 1

Questions

1	Pre-operative investigations	3
2	Problems with medication	5
3	Microbiology	7
4	Antibiotics	9
5	Use of local anaesthesic agents	11
6	Biopsy	13
7	Sterilisation and disinfection	15
8	Sutures	17
9	Wound infection	19
10	Complications of abdominal laparoscopic surgery	21

Question 1:
Theme: Pre-operative investigations

Options:

    a ECG
    b Blood amylase
    c Clotting studies
    d Urine microscopy
    e Random blood glucose
    f Echocardiogram
    g Sickle cell screen

For each of the patients described below, select the single most likely investigation from the options listed above. Each option may be used once, more than once or not at all.

1. A 13-year-old African-Caribbean boy presents to the Accident and Emergency Department with right iliac fossa pain. On examination he has rebound tenderness and guarding in that area. A diagnosis of appendicitis is made and he is scheduled for an emergency appendicectomy.

2. A 48-year-old heavy smoker with a 1-year history of intermittent claudication in his right calf is on the list for an elective right inguinal hernia repair.

3. A 37-year-old non-smoking obese Caucasian woman, whom you are preclerking for an elective cholecystectomy.

Question 1: Answers

1 – g
One must always exclude sickle cell disease in patients of Afro-Caribbean origin in any pre-operative situation.

2 – a
Patients with peripheral vascular disease secondary to atheroma are likely to have similar arterial disease elsewhere. An ECG is a simple and essential test for the investigation of coronary disease.

3 – e
In the West, non-insulin-dependent diabetes mellitus is classically seen in the middle-aged obese population. One must exclude those at risk of being an overt or latent diabetic.

Question 2:
Theme: Problems with medication

Options:

     a Warfarin
     b Thyroxine
     c Captopril
     d Phenytoin
     e Ibuprofen
     f Omeprazole
     g Temazepam
     h Metformin

For each of the situations described below, select the single medication that is contraindicated from the options listed above. Each option may be used once, more than once or not at all.

1. A 23-year-old woman with asthma.

2. A 31-year-old woman with renal artery stenosis.

3. A patient is unable to receive an intravenous urogram if they are taking this medication.

Question 2: Answers

1 – e

Non-steroidal anti-inflammatory drugs block the production of prostaglandins by inhibiting the enzyme cyclo-oxygenase. If this occurs, the metabolites of arachidonic acid are converted to leukotrienes that produce bronchoconstriction and can therefore exacerbate asthma.

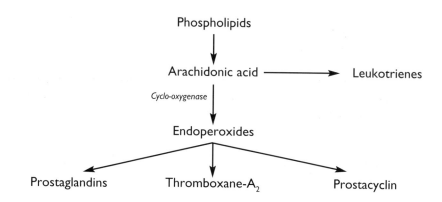

2 – c

Captopril is contraindicated in renal artery stenosis. This condition occurs in **young** women with fibromuscular hyperplasia, or the **elderly** with atherosclerosis. ACE inhibitors such as captopril should not be used in renal artery stenosis as in this disorder maintenance of the renin–angiotensin pathway is critical for adequate renal blood flow.

3 – h

Contraindications to an intravenous urogram are:

- Metformin therapy
- Allergy to seafood and iodine
- Previous allergic reaction to intravenous contrast medium
- Pregnancy

Question 3:
Theme: Microbiology

Options:
- a   *Clostridium tetani*
- b   *Streptococcus pyogenes*
- c   *Staphylococcus aureus*
- d   *Streptococcus faecalis*
- e   *Escherichia coli*
- f   *Clostridium perfringens*

For each of the clinical vignettes described below, select the single most likely pathogen from the options listed above. Each option may be used once, more than once or not at all.

1. A 24-year-old woman complains of a 1-day history of dysuria, haematuria and frequency.

2. A 35-year-old man on the ward complains of headache, stiff jaw muscles, restlessness and wound pain 6 days after sustaining an open fracture of his radius and ulna.

3. A 17-year-old man complains of a red and tender wound 3 days after the removal of a perforated, gangrenous appendix.

4. A 46-year-old man becomes progressively unresponsive over 3 h. On examination he is shocked, pyrexial and has a 1 cm dusky purple discoloured area of his scrotal skin. He can not provide a history revealing how he may have injured his scrotum.

Question 3: Answers

1 – e

The most likely cause of a urinary tract infection in a young previously fit woman is *E. coli*. Other common pathogens include *Proteus mirabilis, Staphylococcus saprophyticus, Staph. epidermidis* and *Enterococcus faecalis*.

2 – a

The likely pathogen is *Clostridium tetani*. The clostridia are spore-forming Gram-positive obligate anaerobes found in human and animal faeces. Their prolonged survival in soil makes dirty wounds prone to infection. Open fractures, which often result in devitalized muscle, are particularly vulnerable.

Clostridium tetani produces two exotoxins: tetanospasmin, a neurotoxin, and tetanolysin, a haemolysin. The former, acting solely on the CNS, is responsible for the clinical features. The prodrome of headache, stiff jaw muscles, risus sardonicus, wound pain and yawning typically occurs after an incubation of 1–2 weeks. This period can vary from between 1 day and 2 months after injury. **The shorter the incubation period, the poorer the prognosis**.

3 – e

Any operation on a perforated bowel has an increased risk of wound infection. The commonest bowel commensals to infect wounds are Gram-negative bacilli and anaerobes. Remember *Streptococcus faecalis* is Gram-positive.

4 – b

This man had necrotizing fasciitis of the scrotum, otherwise known as Fournier's gangrene. The most likely pathogen is *Streptococcus pyogenes* (Lancefield Group A β-haemolytic streptococci). Treatment is wide surgical excision, high-dose intravenous penicillin and appropriate systemic support.

Question 4:
Theme: Antibiotics

Options:

      a   Penicillin
      b   Metronidazole
      c   Flucloxacillin
      d   Co-amoxiclav
      e   Gentamicin

For each of the scenarios described below, select the single most appropriate antibiotic from the options listed above. Each option may be used once, more than once or not at all.

1. An 18-year-old man arrives in the Accident & Emergency Department with a laceration over his fourth right metacarpophalangeal joint sustained when he punched his brother in the mouth.

2. A 78-year-old man presents acutely with confusion and retention of urine. You wish to pass a urinary catheter.

3. A 71-year-old woman recovering from a postoperative urinary tract infection is treated with ciprofloxacin. She subsequently develops fever, abdominal cramps and diarrhoea.

Question 4: Answers

1 – d

The human mouth contains both aerobic and anaerobic organisms that may cause severe infection. It is important to give prophylactic antibiotics as well as to immunize appropriately against tetanus. Check hepatitis B status and arrange HIV counselling and testing if necessary.

2 – e

Intramuscular gentamicin is given before insertion of a urinary catheter as prophylaxis against a bacteraemia caused by traumatic placement of the catheter. Only a **single** dose is needed as antibiotic cover for this procedure.

3 – b

This unfortunate woman is suffering from pseudomembranous colitis, caused by *Clostridium difficile*. Infection typically follows use of clindamycin, though **any** antibiotic may be implicated. This may occur either during or up to 6 weeks after cessation of antibiotic treatment.

Diagnosis is made by detection of *Clostridium difficile* toxin in the stool (**not** stool culture). Complications include toxic megacolon and colonic perforation. All patients should be isolated and barrier nursed.

Remember the rule of fives:

- *Clostridium difficile* is carried in 5% of healthy adults
- **Bloody** diarrhoea is seen in 5% of patients
- 500 mg oral metronidazole is given tds as treatment (intravenous if severe)

An alternative antibiotic to metronidazole is vancomycin, but it is more expensive.

Question 5:
Theme: Use of local anaesthetic agents

Options:

    a   0.5% Bupivicaine
    b   1% Lignocaine and 1:200,000 adrenaline
    c   2% Lignocaine
    d   EMLA cream
    e   1% Prilocaine
    f   4% Amethocaine
    g   1% Lignocaine

For each of the patients described below, select the single most likely type of anaesthetic agent from the options listed above. Each option may be used once, more than once or not at all.

1. An 18-year-old man sustains a 5 cm laceration to his occipital scalp when he is hit over the back of the head by a beer bottle. X-ray reveals no glass in the wound.

2. A 50-year-old builder sustains a closed fracture to his distal radius due to a piece of scaffolding falling onto his forearm. Your registrar has asked you to prepare him for a Bier's block.

3. A 26-year-old woman requires an epidural anaesthetic for an elective Caesarean section.

4. A 57-year-old smoker has a cardiac arrest. ECG monitoring shows ventricular fibrillation. Three loops of CPR have been performed unsuccessfully.

Question 5: Answers

1 – b

Adrenaline is a peripheral vasoconstrictor (acting upon α_1-receptors of the sympathetic nervous system). For this reason it must never be used in end arteries, such as in the digits or in the penis. Vasoconstriction helps to create a bloodless field (very useful in the highly vascular scalp) and enables the anaesthetic to last longer. One may also use a larger maximum dose of anaesthetic, as less is carried away. It therefore lasts longer.

2 – e

Prilocaine is the least cardiotoxic local anaesthetic agent. Bupivicaine has a high affinity for cardiac myocytes, a property that makes it too dangerous to use in intravenous blocks, such as a Bier's block.

3 – a

Bupivicaine (Marcain) is preferred in situations where a long duration of anaesthesia is required. It is commonly used in epidural anaesthesia. Bupivicaine lasts 2–3 h as opposed to the 1–2 h of lignocaine. However, it takes up to 30 min to reach maximum effect.

All local anaesthetics affect the smallest nerve fibres first. As sensory nerve fibres are smaller than motor nerve fibres, a lower concentration (e.g. 0.18%) of bupivicaine will allow the patient to walk even though she has lost sensation in the areas affected by the block. The greater muscle relaxation of 0.5% bupivicaine is useful for the surgery of Caesarean section.

4 – g

Lignocaine has cardiac myocyte membrane-stabilizing properties.

Amethocaine is a topical anaesthetic used in ophthalmology.

EMLA cream is a mixture of topical lignocaine and prilocaine.

Question 6:
Theme: Biopsy

Options:

  a   Fine needle aspiration
  b   Core biopsy
  c   Brush cytology
  d   Crosby capsule
  e   Endoscopic biopsy
  f   Surgical excision

For each of the clinical case scenarios described below, select the single most likely method of biopsy from the options listed above. Each option may be used once, more than once or not at all.

1. A 41-year-old woman presents with agitation, palpitations and a lump in her throat that moves up on swallowing.

2. A 25-year-old woman attends her general practitioner for a routine cervical smear.

3. A 71-year-old man notices a lump on his nose. On examination, it is a 1 cm pearly pink papule with a few overlying telangiectases. It has a rolled edge.

4. A 62-year-old woman has jaundice, weight loss and an enlarged liver. CT scan of the abdomen reveals a solid mass in the liver.

Question 6: Answers

1 – a
Fine-needle aspiration cytology (FNAC) is particularly useful in diagnosing breast and thyroid lumps. A common pitfall often asked in multiple choice questions is that FNAC can be used to distinguish between **papillary** adenoma and carcinoma, but not between **follicular** adenoma and carcinoma. **Histology** is needed to show whether the capsule has been invaded for follicular carcinoma, and hence FNAC is not adequate as it demonstrates **cytology** only.

2 – c
Brush cytology is used in this screening process. The pathologist does not need to look at the cervical **architecture** (histology), only the actual cells (cytology).

3 – f
A basal cell carcinoma needs removal, with a 0.5 cm margin, as it is a slow growing, typically non-metastasizing tumour. A squamous cell carcinoma requires margins of 1 cm at removal. The resection margins of malignant melanoma depends on the stage (see page 98).

4 – b
Core biopsies such as Tru-Cut, Surecut, Biopty and drill biopsies are used when cytoarchitecture is required for diagnosis. They are useful for solid lesions, for example, liver, breast and sarcoma.

Question 7:
Theme: Sterilisation and disinfection

Options:

    a   γ-irradiation
    b   Ethylene oxide
    c   Steam/pressure sterilization
    d   Low temperature steam and formaldehyde
    e   Hot air
    f   Boiling water
    g   Glutaraldehyde
    h   Little Sister autoclave

For each of the materials described below, select the single most likely method of sterilisation from the options listed above. Each option may be used once, more than once or not at all.

1. Disinfection of endoscopes.

2. Sterilisation of flexible–fibre endoscopes.

3. Drill bit dropped during dynamic hip screw insertion.

Question 7: Answers

1 – g

Disinfection **reduces** the number of viable micro-organisms. Some viruses and bacterial spores may be left active. This is different to sterilisation, which is the **complete** destruction or removal of all viable micro-organisms, including spores and viruses.

2 – b

Ethylene oxide is an effective sterilisation agent, but it is also flammable, toxic, irritant and potentially carcinogenic! As it is flammable, it can only be used to sterilise heat-sensitive materials.

3 – h

A Little Sister autoclave, a portable steam steriliser, is ideal for a dropped instrument as it is much quicker than a pressure steam autoclave. Remember that any blood needs to be washed off first to stop it getting caked on the instrument.

Question 8:
Theme: Sutures

Options:
- a   PDS (polydiaxone)
- b   Vicryl (polyglactin)
- c   Prolene (polypropylene)
- d   PTFE (polytetrafluoroethylene)
- e   Metal clips
- f   Catgut
- g   Silk

For each of the wounds described below, select the single most likely suture material from the options listed above. Each option may be used once, more than once or not at all.

1.   A 19-year-old man is punched in the face. His tooth lacerates the mucosa on the inside of his lower lip. He has requested an absorbable suture.

2.   Suturing tensor fascia lata post total hip replacement.

3.   Suturing the anastomosis of a femoro-popliteal bypass graft.

Question 8: Answers

1 – f
Catgut

2 – b
Vicryl

3 – c
Prolene

Suture	Type	Tensile strength	Absorption time
Plain catgut	Absorbable monofil	21 days	90 days
Chromic catgut	Absorbable monofil	28 days	90 days
PDS	Absorbable monofil	56 days	180 days
Vicryl	Absorbable braided	30 days	60–90 days
Prolene	Non-absorbable monofil	Indefinite	Non-absorbable
Silk	Non-absorbable, braided	1 year	2 years
Metal clips	n/a	Indefinite	Non-absorbable

PTFE coats braided synthetic suture material to smooth the material and to decrease capillary action, e.g. Ethiflex.

Question 9:
Theme: Wound infection

Options:
- a   Clean
- b   Clean–contaminated
- c   Contaminated
- d   Dirty

For each of the operations described below, select the single most likely category from the options listed above. Each option may be used once, more than once or not at all.

1. Appendicectomy on a 15-year-old girl with a perforated appendix.

2. An uncomplicated elective right hemicolectomy in a 61-year-old man.

3. Repair of a direct inguinal hernia in a 31-year-old man.

Question 9: Answers

1 – d
See the table for an explanation.

2 – c
As above.

3 – a
As above.

Category	Example	Percentage infected
Clean	Incisions through non-infected skin that do not breach any hollow organ, e.g. inguinal hernia repair	1.5
Clean–contaminated	Incisions that breach a hollow viscus other than the colon, e.g. open cholecystectomy	< 8
Contaminated	Incisions contaminated by opening the colon, open fractures or animal/human bites	12
Dirty	Wounds made in the presence of pus, a perforated viscus or traumatic wounds of > 4 h duration	25

Question 10:
Theme: Complications of abdominal laparoscopic surgery

Options:

 a Inferior epigastric artery tear
 b Pneumonia
 c Myocardial infarction
 d Abdominal aorta tear
 e Right hepatic artery tear
 f Perforated viscus
 g Air embolism

For each of the patients described below, select the single most likely complication from the options listed above. Each option may be used once, more than once or not at all.

1. A 45-year-old man complains of increasingly severe abdominal pain 8 h after an elective laparoscopic left inguinal hernia repair. On examination, he is sweaty, tachycardic and apyrexial. His abdomen is rigid with rebound, guarding and absent bowel sounds.

2. While performing your first laparoscopic cholecystectomy, the anaesthetist advises you that the patient is becoming increasingly tachycardic, and the latest blood pressure is lowered at 100/70 mmHg. You note a 5 cm soft, purple, subcutaneous abdominal mass extending from your second port of entry site.

Question 10: Answers

1 – f

It is safer to introduce the first trochar after opening the peritoneum with a scalpel under direct vision (this is the method to learn for exam purposes and future practice). However, blind insertion of the first trochar of laparoscopy is still commonly undertaken. With the latter technique it has been known for the bowel to be nicked without anything being noticed until the patient can tell you so! Similar perforation of the aorta will be a lot more catastrophic and easier to see when a laparosocope is introduced into the peritoneal cavity. Hence, to maintain a good pneumoperitoneum, push the trochar with slow, even pressure, holding your fingers near the tip of the trochar to prevent it slipping too far. The patient is head down and one aims towards the pelvis in the midline to avoid the bowel and aorta, which bifurcates at the level of the fourth lumbar vertebra.

2 – a

The inferior epigastric artery has a very variable course, originating from the femoral artery and running superficial to the rectus abdominis in between the linea semilunaris laterally and the linea alba medially. If not stemmed, the patient can exsanguinate from such a wound. There is no failsafe way to avoid it (ultrasound of the abdomen while inserting a trochar is not feasible), but going through the linea semilunaris is a safe bet!

Core Module 2: Peri-operative Management 2

Questions

1	Surgical dressings	25
2	Acid-base balance	27
3	Nutrition	29
4	Anaemia	31
5	Bleeding disorders	33
6	Postoperative shortness of breath	35
7	Postoperative pyrexia	37
8	Postoperative nerve palsies	39
9	Analgesia	41
10	Infection in the immunocompromised patient	43

Question 1:
Theme: Surgical dressings

Options:

- a   Intrasite gel and gauze
- b   No dressing
- c   Gelonet
- d   Elastoplast
- e   Antiseptic-impregnated paraffin gauze dressing
- f   Polyurethane incise drape

For each of the wounds described below, select the single most likely dressing from the options listed above. Each option may be used once, more than once or not at all.

1.   A 36-year-old housewife accidentally pours a mug of hot coffee over her wrist. Examination reveals a partial thickness burn.

2.   A 83-year-old man has chronic venous leg ulcers.

3.   A 40-year-old man has a pilonidal abscess; it has been widely excised, and has a sloughy cavity base.

Question I: Answers

1 – e

Occlusive dressings prevent bacterial entry causing infection. Paraffin helps to prevent leakage, which would present external environment bacteria with a direct path to the wound ('strike-through'). Maintaining a moist environment aids native tissue debriding necrotic material and promotes healing.

2 – c

Venous leg ulcers typically take a long time to heal due to the debilitated nature of the patient. Sheet polymeric dressings are used for these superficial open wounds. These may be a **hydrocolloid** (e.g. granuflex – a fully occlusive dressing) or **hydrogels** (e.g. the semi-occlusive geliperm). All draw out the slough of the wound and prevent excess exudate by their high absorbency. Kaltostat or Sorban act in a similar manner, but are not occlusive on their own and are distinguished by having a biological source – algae – hence the term 'alginates', and are used for bleeding wounds and heavily exuding wounds.

3 – a

Intrasite gel is a hydrogel and is used to draw out the slough of (especially cavitated) wounds. It contains activated charcoal and is therefore useful for malodorous wounds. If the wound floor is clean and granulating, some may advocate the use of (expensive) silicone foam dressings such as 'cavicare' that expand to fill the wound space.

Type of wound	Type of dressing
Bleeding wounds	Alginates (e.g. Kaltostat)
Lightly exuding wounds	Hydrocolloid sheet (e.g. granuflex)
Heavily exuding wounds	Alginates covered with an absorbent pad
Infected wounds	Intrasite gel ± antibiotic
Offensively smelling wounds	Intrasite gel containing activated charcoal
Cavitated wounds	Alginate packing; silastic foam
Necrotic or sloughy wounds	Intrasite gel; Debrizan paste

Wound dressing usage differs widely across the profession, partly due to a lack of satisfactory clinical trials, good advertising and economics.

Question 2:
Theme: Acid-base balance

Options:

    a   Panic attack
    b   Diabetic ketoacidosis
    c   Exacerbation of chronic obstructive pulmonary disease
    d   Hyperemesis gravidarum

For each of the blood gas results described below, select the single most likely condition from the options listed above. Each option may be used once, more than once or not at all.

	pH	HCO_3^- (mmol/l)	pCO_2 (kPa)	pO_2 (kPa)
1.	7.25	35	10.0	8.6
2.	7.19	8	2.9	14.0
3.	7.55	41	6.2	11.7

Question 2: Answers

1 – c

Respiratory acidosis. A low respiratory rate will not 'blow off' CO_2 and therefore the CO_2 will form HCO_3^- causing acidosis. The cause is respiratory.

2 – b

Metabolic acidosis. In DKA, lack of insulin prevents glucose entering cells to be metabolised. Energy is therefore derived from fat lipolysis, which breaks down fats into ketones in the mitochondria. Ketones are acidic and accumulate. The cause is metabolic.

3 – d

Metabolic alkalosis. Severe vomiting makes one lose large amounts of H^+ ions from the stomach, causing alkalosis. The cause is metabolic.

We found that the acid-base balance is explained comprehensively in the STEP course reader. However, we find the following regimen useful when looking at blood gas results:

- Look at the pH. Is the patient acidotic or alkalotic? You have now done half the question.
- Look at the HCO_3^- and the pCO_2. One will be **much** more abnormal than the other. If the pCO_2 is the more abnormal, then the problem is respiratory; if the HCO_3^- is the more abnormal then the problem is metabolic.

Remember that pO_2 **should** be very high if the patient is on oxygen. Do not be lulled into a false sense of security by a **normal** oxygen value on such a patient.

Normal values for arterial blood gases:
- pH = 7.35–7.45
- PaO_2 = > 10.6 kPa
- $PaCO_2$ = 4.7–6.0 kPa
- HCO_3^- = 24–30 mmol/l

Question 3:
Theme: Nutrition

Options:

    a   Total parenteral nutrition
    b   Oral elemental diet
    c   Percutaneous endoscopic gastrostomy (PEG)
    d   Nasojejunostomy
    e   Needle catheter jejunostomy (NCJ)
    f   Nasogastric feeding

For each of the clinical vignettes described below, select the single most likely method of feeding from the options listed above. Each option may be used once, more than once or not at all.

1. A 69-year-old man presented with significant weight loss and change in bowel habit. A mass was felt per rectum and he underwent a difficult abdomino-perineal resection, with some faecal contamination peri-operatively. He has not passed flatus since the operation. Recovery is anticipated to take a long time.

2. A 72-year-old woman suffered a left-sided cerebrovascular accident during an elective abdominal aortic aneurysm repair. Four weeks later she still has no gag reflex. It is anticipated that she will be unable to feed herself for some time.

3. A 71-year-old man suffers increasing dysphagia over some months. He has a lower oesophageal carcinoma. It proves impossible to pass a nasogastric tube. His is malnourished, and it is decided that he will need nutritional support before surgery.

Question 3: Answers

1 – a

2 – c

3 – e

Just as more potent analgesics can be given according to severity of pain as dictated by the analgesic ladder, the provision of nutrition may also be looked upon as following a 'nutritional ladder'.

Enteral diets are always more preferable to parenteral ones; they use and therefore increase the blood supply to the GI tract. This will then remain intact and will not allow the bacteria inside it to translocate to the bloodstream. If the gut is working, an enteral diet is used.

Enteral diets may be given orally or via a tube. The standard diet is called a polymeric diet. If the function of the patient's gut is decreased but still capable of absorbing the basic nutrients, then a **predigested** or **elemental** diet may be used. This may be enough to induce remission in mild cases of inflammatory bowel disease.

An oral diet is given whenever possible. In those patients who require nutritional support for < 4 weeks, the diet may be given by a fine-bore nasogastric tube instead, or as well as the oral diet. If there is **gastric** stasis (as will happen commonly in critically ill or post-surgical patients), then the tube needs to be pushed past the pylorus into the duodenum or jejunum, thereby instigating **nasoduodenal** or **-jejunal** feeding and preventing aspiration pneumonia.

For patients requiring > 4 weeks of feeding, it is necessary to introduce a tube into the gut surgically. This may be a PEG, which is the treatment of choice in most cases. It is also possible to use an NCJ, which is distal to the duodenum and will therefore allow feeding after major upper GI surgery.

Those patients who have non-functioning bowels will require parenteral nutrition.

Question 4:
Theme: Anaemia

Options:
- a   Carcinoma of the stomach
- b   Crohn's disease
- c   Pernicious anaemia
- d   Carcinoma of the breast
- e   Carcinoma of the caecum
- f   Haemorrhoids
- g   Diverticular disease

For each of the patients described below, select the single most likely diagnosis from the options listed above. Each option may be used once, more than once or not at all.

1. A 52-year-old woman presents with shortness of breath. She has no significant past medical history. Investigations reveal iron deficiency anaemia, but she has no specific symptoms and a normal gastroscopy.

2. A 32-year-old woman presents with signs and symptoms of bowel obstruction. She has had previous similar attacks over the past 8 months, with some weight loss. She gives a history of bowel resection in her early teens. Her Hb = 9.0 g/dl with a MCV = 112.

3. A 70-year-old woman complains of fatigue and lethargy. On examination she has a swelling in her left armpit. She refuses further examination. She has a leuco-erythroblastic anaemia on her peripheral blood film.

Question 4: Answers

1 – e

Carcinoma of the caecum often results in silent bleeding and therefore iron loss. Patients will subsequently present with signs and symptoms of iron deficiency anaemia.

2 – b

Crohn's disease affects the terminal ileum more than anywhere else in the GI tract. Vitamin B_{12} is absorbed here, and its deficiency causes a megaloblastic anaemia.

3 – d

On a peripheral blood film, a leuco-erythroblastic anaemia is seen as the presence of immature cells (myelocytes and normoblasts). It is due to bone marrow infiltration, in this case due to malignancy, but may also occur secondary to hypoxia or any severe anaemia.

Question 5:
Theme: Bleeding disorders

Options:

a   Haemophilia
b   Von Willebrand's disease
c   Warfarin therapy
d   Heparin therapy
e   Disseminated intravascular coagulation
f   Protein C deficiency
g   Autoimmune thrombocytopaenia
h   Essential thrombocythaemia

For each of the sets of investigations described below, select the single most likely diagnosis from the options listed above. Each option may be used once, more than once or not at all.

1   INR = 3.0   APTT = 2.5   TT = 1.5
    Hb = 9.7 g/dl   WCC = 15.8 × 10^9/l   plt = 60 × 10^9/l

2   INR = 1.1   APTT = 1.0   TT = 1.1
    Hb = 14.0 g/dl   WCC = 8.0 × 10^9/l   plt = 25 × 10^9/l

INR, international normalized ratio; APTT, activated partial thrombin time; TT, thrombin time; Hb, haemoglobin; WCC, white cell count; plt, platelet count.

Question 5: Answers

1 – e

DIC is an uncontrolled activation of the fibrinolytic and coagulation pathways. For the exam, remember DIC is when everything goes up except for Hb and platelets, which go down!

2 – g

Autoimmune thrombocytopaenia is suspected when the platelet count is very low, but all other tests are normal.

- **INR** is a ratio of the patient's **PT** to control and tests the **extrinsic** system
- **APTT** = PTTK = KCCT = PTT and tests the **intrinsic** system
- Warfarin antagonizes vitamin K, inhibiting action of factors II, VII, IX and X. Early warfarin therapy thus prolongs PT alone, whereas full warfarinisation prolongs PT and APTT. It is tested by measuring INR
- Heparin inhibits the action of thrombin and potentiates anti-thrombin III. Heparin anticoagulation is tested by measuring APTT
- Haemophilia is an X-linked deficiency of factors VIII (haemophilia A) or IX (haemophilia B). Both factors form part of the intrinsic pathway. Their deficiency therefore will result in a prolonged APTT

Look up the clotting cascade while reading the above and check your understanding using the table below:

PT	APTT	TT	Plt	BT*	Cause
↑	↔	↔	↔	↔	**Extrinsic system**: early warfarin therapy; factor VII deficiency
↔	↑	↔	↔	↔	**Intrinsic system**: heparin; haemophilia;
↔	↑	↔	↔	↑	VW disease
↑	↑	↑	↓	↑	**Common pathway**: DIC; acute liver disease
↔	↔	↔	↔	↔	Platelet function disorder
↑	↑	↔	↔	↔	Vitamin K deficiency; warfarin

*BT, bleeding time

Question 6:
Theme: Postoperative shortness of breath

Options:
- a Acute bronchopneumonia post-atelectasis
- b Pulmonary embolism
- c ARDS
- d Pneumothorax
- e Gastric aspiration
- f Heart failure
- g Hyperventilation

For each of the clinical vignettes described below, select the single most likely diagnosis from the options listed above. Each option may be used once, more than once or not at all.

1. A 35-year-old woman undergoes an open cholecystectomy. She complains of pain from the wound site after the operation, which is poorly treated. The pain is so severe that she is not compliant with her chest physiotherapy. After 3 days she becomes pyrexial with a productive cough. A chest X-ray reveals left lower lobe consolidation.

2. A 68-year-old woman undergoes a right hip replacement for severe osteoarthritis. Three days postoperatively she suddenly collapses after walking back from the toilet. On examination, her airway is clear. Her respiratory rate = 26 breaths min^{-1}; O$_2$ saturation = 75% on air. Chest examination is surprisingly unremarkable and an ECG shows sinus tachycardia only.

3. A 16-year-old girl undergoes an appendicectomy. She is known to have cystic fibrosis.

4. A 62-year-old man undergoes a reversal of Hartmann's procedure. Two days later he becomes unwell and pyrexial, with a rigid and tender abdomen. He then undergoes a laparotomy to repair his leaking anastomosis. Twenty-four hours later he becomes tachycardic and tachypnoeic, and 1 day later he is hypoxaemic despite oxygen therapy. Chest examination reveals a few inspiratory rhonchi with a normal chest X-ray.

Question 6: Answers

1 – a

If breathing is painful, as may occur after upper abdominal or any thoracic surgery, then the patient is less willing to cough up mucus. This will then plug up the small airways, which will collapse distally, producing atelectasis. Superinfection will result in pneumonia. A CXR may show lobar consolidation.

2 – b

Deep vein thrombosis and therefore pulmonary embolism is much more likely after orthopaedic or pelvic surgery. It must always be borne in mind when a patient becomes tachycardic or dyspnoeic postoperatively. There may be a paucity of signs, especially if the patient is on oxygen when you arrive.

3 – d

This is a recognized complication of cystic fibrosis.

4 – c

It is difficult to define ARDS, but it may be thought of as non-cardiogenic pulmonary oedema, precipitated by many different conditions and causing hypoxia. As the pulmonary oedema is non-cardiogenic, it may be differentiated from cardiogenic pulmonary oedema by a normal or low left atrial pressure. It may be divided into four stages:

- Up to 24 h post-insult – tachycardia and tachypnoea only
- Up to 48 h post-insult – may be a few inspiratory rhonchi; hypoxaemia despite O_2 therapy
- Following phase 2 – high pitched inspiratory rhonchi; chest X-ray shows bilateral diffuse lung infiltration
- Following phase 3 – lethargy, coma, multiple organ failure

The best treatment involves a high index of clinical suspicion, thus preventing progression.

Question 7:
Theme: Postoperative pyrexia

Options:
- a   Bronchopneumonia
- b   Transfusion reaction
- c   Deep vein thrombosis
- d   Urinary tract infection
- e   Infection of intravenous cannula site
- f   Superficial wound infection
- g   Allergic drug reaction

For each of the clinical vignettes described below, select the single most likely diagnosis from the options listed above. Each option may be used once, more than once or not at all.

1. A 61-year-old man undergoes a Whipple's procedure to remove a pancreatic carcinoma. He is unwilling to get out of bed after the operation. Five days later he develops a low-grade fever and a swollen, tender right calf.

2. A 63-year-old woman develops a pyrexia 6 days after her abdominal aortic aneurysm repair. She is systemically well. While measuring her central venous pressure you note that her neck appears to be red and hot.

Question 7: Answers

1 – c
This is a classic presentation of a DVT.

2 – e
This is most likely to be infection of her central venous catheter, which has been left unchanged for 6 days.

Question 8:
Theme: Postoperative nerve palsies

Options:

    a   Common peroneal nerve
    b   Recurrent laryngeal nerve
    c   External laryngeal nerve
    d   Facial nerve
    e   Spinal accessory nerve
    f   Phrenic nerve

For each of the operations described below, select the single most likely nerve palsy from the options listed above. Each option may be used once, more than once or not at all.

1. A 38-year-old woman undergoes a subtotal thyroidectomy. After operation she notices that she can no longer sing the high notes while in her church choir.

2. A 28-year-old man has a lump in the posterior part of his neck removed as a daycase. After operation he notices that he has difficulty shrugging the shoulder on that side.

3. A 44-year-old woman post total vaginal hysterectomy.

Question 8: Answers

1 – c

Every muscle in the larynx is supplied by the recurrent laryngeal nerve, **except** for cricothyroid, which is supplied by the external laryngeal nerve. Both are branches of the vagus nerve. Cricothyroid is used to stretch the vocal cords, which increases vocal pitch. Its paralysis results in a pair of slack cords that struggle to produce high notes.

Recurrent laryngeal nerve palsy causes the vocal cord on that side to remain abducted, producing a gap between the cords. This will produce a breathy voice and a bovine cough, which typically worsens as the day progresses. This is because the vocal cord that comes across to fill the gap fatigues through the day.

See also page 158.

2 – e

The spinal accessory nerve runs across the posterior triangle of the neck. Its surface marking is from one-third of the way down sternomastoid to one-third of the way up trapezius. The patient therefore has a paralysed trapezius.

Occasionally, the unsuspecting SHO will damage the spinal accessory nerve while removing a lump in the neck.

3 – a

This patient was placed in the lithotomy position. The pressure from the leg support bar pressed against the neck of her fibula, which is the surface marking for the common peroneal nerve. As its deep peroneal branch supplies the ankle dorsiflexors she will have a foot drop on that side when she wakes up.

Question 9:
Theme: Analgesia

Options:
    a   Paracetamol
    b   1% Lignocaine
    c   Carbamazepine
    d   Diclofenac sodium
    e   Glyceryl trinitrate
    f   Nitrous oxide
    g   Diamorphine
    h   1% Lignocaine with 1:200,000 adrenaline

For each of the clinical scenarios described below, select the single most likely analgesic from the options listed above. Each option may be used once, more than once or not at all.

1. A 29-year-old woman with trigeminal neuralgia.

2. A 37-year-old man with left–sided renal colic.

3. A 41-year-old woman requiring drainage of a paronychia on her right index finger.

Question 9: Answers

1 – c

If medication is unsuccessful, it is possible either percutaneously to thermocoagulate or even perform microvascular decompression of the fifth cranial nerve using Dandy's posterior fossa approach.

2 – d

This medication is often introduced rectally. Buscopan (hyoscine butylbromide) is a useful antispasmodic also usually given. If the patient is still in pain, opiates may then be used.

3 – b

This patient requires a digital nerve ring block before incision and drainage of her paronychia. If a mixture containing adrenaline is used, this will induce vasoconstriction of the digital arteries. As these are end arteries, the finger will become avascular and therefore gangrenous.

Question 10:
Theme: Infection in the immunocompromised patient

Options:

  a *Pneumocystis carinii* pneumonia
  b Pulmonary tuberculosis
  c *Cryptosporidium*
  d *Toxoplasmosis gondii*
  e Candidiasis
  f Herpes simplex virus
  g *Pseudomonas aeruginosa*

For each of the patients described below, select the single most likely organism from the options listed above. Each option may be used once, more than once or not at all.

1. A 31-year-old HIV-positive man suffers from progressively worsening diarrhoea and weight loss over the past 3 weeks.

2. A 29-year-old intravenous drug abuser has been admitted for treatment of his injection site cellulitis. While on the ward his dry cough becomes worse, and is now accompanied by dyspnoea and pyrexia. CXR reveals bilateral pulmonary interstitial infiltrates.

3. A 41-year-old woman has an active thyroid nodule for which she is on carbimazole therapy before surgery. She develops a fever and a productive cough. A Gram stain of her sputum contains Gram-negative bacilli.

Question 10: Answers

1 – c

Cryptosporidium is the commonest cause of severe diarrhoea in patients infected with HIV. It is diagnosed by microscopy of either a stool sample or by intestinal biopsy.

No therapeutic agent is completely efficacious against this protozoan, and treatment is therefore largely supportive. Patients are advised to drink boiled water as the organism is heat-sensitive.

2 – a

This particular patient was infected with HIV as a result of his drug habit. There are often few clinical signs on chest examination in patients infected with PCP.

First-line treatment is with co-trimoxazole.

Second-line treatment is with clindamycin and primaquine, or dapsone and trimethoprim.

Glucocorticoids may be added for severe infections (PaO_2 < 8.2 kPa on air).

3 – g

Carbimazole produces leucopaenia or skin rashes in ~1% of patients, usually in the first 6 weeks of treatment. Neutropaenic patients are especially susceptible to infection by Gram-negative organisms, but Gram-positive infections are becoming more frequent.

Core Module 3: Trauma

Questions

1	Diagnosis in primary survey	47
2	Hypovolaemic shock	49
3	Head injury	51
4	Glasgow Coma Score	53
5	Traumatic injury of the peripheral nervous system	55
6	Fracture management	57
7	Complications of fractures	59
8	Spinal injuries	61
9	Tendon anatomy and injury	63
10	Burns	65

Question 1:
Theme: Diagnosis in primary survey

Options:

    a   Tension pneumothorax
    b   Cardiac tamponade
    c   Flail segment
    d   Subdural haematoma
    e   Massive haemothorax
    f   Ruptured spleen
    g   Ruptured thoracic aorta

For each of the patients described below, select the single most likely diagnosis from the options listed above. Each option may be used once, more than once or not at all.

1. A 25-year-old man drinks several pints of beer in his local pub, and drives into a tree at 40 mph on his way home. On arrival at the Accident and Emergency Department he is in obvious distress. Vital signs are BP = 90/40, heart rate = 150 min^{-1}, RR = 45 min^{-1}. His neck veins are distended. On examination of the chest the heart sounds are faint and the trachea is central.

2. A 31-year-old pedestrian is hit by a passing motorcycle as she crosses the road. She complains of abdominal and chest pain. On examination BP = 86/32, heart rate = 145 min^{-1}. She has bruising and tenderness over her lower left ninth and tenth ribs. She has rebound tenderness and guarding over the left upper quadrant of her abdomen.

Question 1: Answers

1 – b
A patient with a cardiac tamponade will classically exhibit Beck's triad:

- Quiet, muffled heart sounds
- Hypotension
- A raised JVP on inspiration (Kussmaul's sign)

2 – f
The woman is likely to have suffered a ruptured spleen. This is usually given away by the fact that there is a rib fracture of the left-sided ninth-to-eleventh ribs with concomitant hypotension. A later sign will be purple mottling of the skin over the left upper quadrant of the abdomen from haemorrhage.

Facts about the spleen conveniently fall into the 'odd numbers rule'. The spleen is $1 \times 3 \times 5$ inches in dimension, 7 oz in mass and lies beneath the ninth-to-eleventh ribs.

Question 2:
Theme: Hypovolaemic shock

Options:

        a   Grade 1
        b   Grade 2
        c   Grade 3
        d   Grade 4

For each of the sets of vital signs described below, select the single most likely grade of shock from the options listed above. Each option may be used once, more than once or not at all.

	Heart rate (beats min^{-1})	Pulse pressure (mmHg)	Urine output (ml h^{-1})	Systolic BP (mmHg)
1.	110	Decreased	30	120
2.	150	Decreased	2	60
3.	95	Normal	45	125

Question 2: Answers

1 – b

2 – d

3 – a

Shock can be defined as inadequate tissue and organ perfusion. In the trauma scenario it is very likely to be due to hypovolaemia. Causes of hypovolaemic shock that must be taken into account are:

Haemorrhage
- an open exsanguinating wound
- a fracture
- massive haemothorax (consider ruptured aorta)
- ruptured spleen/liver
- torn mesenteric artery

Burns

The table is useful to learn for the exam. The blood loss associated with each grade of shock can be remembered as a 'tennis score' system, i.e. grade 1 shock is blood loss of up to 15%, grade 2 shock between 15 and 30%, etc.

	Grade 1	Grade 2	Grade 3	Grade 4
Blood loss (%)	0–15	15–30	30–40	> 40
Heart rate (beats min⁻¹)	< 100	100–120	120–140	> 140
Pulse pressure	Normal	Decreased	Decreased	Decreased
Systolic BP	Normal	Normal	Decreased	Decreased
Urine output (ml h⁻¹)	> 30	20–30	5–15	< 5
Mental state	Alert	Aggressive	Confused	Drowsy/coma
Capillary refill	Normal	Delayed (> 2 s)	Delayed	Absent

It is worth noting that by the time a patient has a lowered systolic blood pressure, they will already have lost at least 30% of their blood volume.

Question 3:
Theme: Head injury

Options:

     a Extradural haematoma
     b Subdural haematoma
     c Intracerebral haematoma
     d Base of skull fracture
     e Le Fort I fracture
     f Le Fort II fracture
     g Le Fort III fracture

For each of the patients described below, select the single most likely pathology from the options listed above. Each option may be used once, more than once or not at all.

1. A 34-year-old man is assaulted by two muggers, one of whom hits him on the side of his head with a baseball bat. On admission his airway is clear, and he is breathing spontaneously. He has bruising behind the mastoid process on his left side, although the bat did not strike this area.

2. An 81-year-old woman trips up at home while walking from the bedroom to the bathroom. Even though she hits her head on the floor, she does not lose consciousness. Her husband calls an ambulance 4 days later as he is worried that she has been slipping in and out of a drowsy state.

3. A 24-year-old man collides with another car at 60 mph. On admission he has blood caked over his face and appears to be in some distress. He is intubated and his vital signs are stabilized during the primary survey. Skull X-ray reveals that he has a fracture extending from the alveolar part of his maxilla to the medial infra-orbital rim, which meets a similar fracture from the other side across the nasal bones.

Question 3: Answers

1 – d

It is important to exclude a base of skull fracture in any head injury. This can manifest itself in the following ways:

- Retromastoid bruising (Battle's sign)
- Bilateral peri-orbital haematoma (Panda eyes sign); also caused by bleeding under the scalp from a 'de-gloving' injury, e.g. a child being pulled by its hair
- CSF otorrhoea ± blood (if blood only is seen, test for sugar which will indicate the presence of CSF, hidden by the blood)
- CSF rhinorrhoea (if bleeding also, 'tramlines' will be seen, where clear CSF washes a track through the centre of the trickle of blood
- Caroticocavernous fistula – a fracture in the middle cranial fossa may tear the internal carotid artery within the cavernous sinus. This will produce a fistula between the two, causing an increase in pressure from the sinus through the ophthalmic veins into the orbit. The patient will complain of a rushing sound in the head and may display a proptosis on one side. There may also be an ophthalmoplegia as a result of impaired third, fourth or sixth cranial nerve dysfunction.

2 – b

This is a classic history of a **sub**dural haematoma. In the elderly, senile brain atrophy creates a larger subdural space, across which bridging veins pass from the cerebral cortex to the sinuses. A fall will shear these veins, thus producing a **venous** bleed that classically manifests itself as a fluctuation in consciousness.

An **extra**dural bleed classically has a very different history. The initiating injury is usually a sharp blow to the side of the head, over the area at which the parietal, frontal, temporal and sphenoid bones meet (the **pterion**). The skull here is particularly thin, and is either in front of or contains the middle meningeal artery. The blow itself will often produce a loss of consciousness, which is transient. Then follows the **lucid interval**, during which time the artery, which is **between** the dura and the skull, bleeds to form a haematoma that peels the dura off its overlying bone.

If large enough, either clot will produce an increase in intracranial pressure large enough to produce neurological symptoms and eventually death. The warning sign of this is an ipsilateral dilated pupil, due to pressure on CN III resulting in the eye losing its parasympathetic input.

3 – f

Le Fort discovered how the mid-**facial** bones fractured by dropping heavy weights onto cadaveric faces. He observed three patterns of injury, which are known as the Le Fort I, II and III fractures. They are produced by a large amount of force; thus particular attention must be paid to the airway.

Question 4:
Theme: Glasgow Coma Score

Options:

a	5
b	6
c	7
d	8
e	9
f	10
g	12
h	14
i	15

For each of the patients described below, select the appropriate Glasgow Coma Scale score from the options listed above. Each option may be used once, more than once or not at all.

1. A 38-year-old woman is hit over the head with an iron bar. She opens her eyes to speech, and talks in a lucid manner. She moves her limbs spontaneously.

2. A 16-year-old boy falls off some scaffolding and lands on his head. On arrival to the Accident and Emergency Department he opens his eyes to pain and makes only grunting noises. He withdraws his limbs from painful stimuli.

3. A 46-year-old man is involved in a high-speed road traffic accident in which he is thrown from the car. He opens his eyes to speech and localizes painful stimuli. He can speak but his sentences sound confused.

Question 4: Answers

1 – h
Motor score = 6
Verbal score = 5
Eye score = 3

2 – d
Motor score = 4
Verbal score = 2
Eye score = 2

3 – g
Motor score = 5
Verbal score = 4
Eye score = 3

The Glasgow Coma Scale (GCS) is an objective measurement of consciousness. It is particularly useful because a change in Glasgow Coma scale is often significant of underlying change in condition of the patient. It has to be learned, as you may well be asked to work out GCS scores in the exam.

The GCS consists of three separate scores, one each for verbal, motor and eye responses. These are added to from a total out of 15. It is impossible to score < 3.

Score	Motor	Verbal	Eye
6	Normal	–	–
5	Localizing to pain	Lucid	–
4	Withdrawing from pain	Confused speech	Eyes open spontaneously
3	Flexion to pain (decorticate)	Words only	Eyes open to speech
2	Extension to pain (decerebrate)	Sounds only	Eyes open to pain
1	No response	No sounds	Eyes do not open

Question 5:
Theme: Traumatic injury of the peripheral nervous system

Options:

  a   Deep branch of the radial nerve
  b   Superficial branch of the radial nerve
  c   Common peroneal nerve
  d   Ulnar nerve at elbow
  e   Ulnar nerve at wrist
  f   Median nerve at elbow
  g   Axillary nerve
  h   Sciatic nerve in the buttock

For each of the observations described below, select the single most likely nerve injury from the options listed above. Each option may be used once, more than once or not at all.

1. A 39-year-old woman trips over while gardening and falls through a greenhouse window, lacerating her outstretched arm. On examination she can not grip a piece of paper between her fingers on that side. There is no clawing of her hand.

2. A 15-year-old boy falls on his shoulder after being tackled during a rugby match. It is noted that he has lost sensation to the skin over the lateral mid-shaft of his humerus.

3. A 21-year-old man is stabbed in the upper part of the forearm with a broken bottle. On examination he can not extend his wrist or fingers. There is no distal sensory deficit.

Question 5: Answers

1 – d

This is an example of the so-called 'ulnar paradox', in which a transection of the ulnar nerve at the **wrist** causes hand clawing but transection higher up at the **elbow** results in much **less** clawing of the hand. The anatomical reason is as follows:

An ulnar nerve injury denervates the ulnar (medial) two lumbricals, which are used to extend the ring and little fingers at the metacapophalangeal joints. Loss of these muscles means that the flexor digitorum muscles can now flex these fingers, causing a clawed appearance.

If the ulnar nerve is cut at the elbow joint, the muscles described above will still be paralysed. However, in the forearm the ulnar nerve gives off a branch to the part of flexor digitorum profundus, which usually flexes the ring and little fingers. As this will no longer be working with a high lesion, there is less flexion of these fingers and the claw is lost.

2 – g

The posterior cord of the brachial plexus splits to form the axillary nerve and the radial nerve. The axillary nerve winds around the back of the humerus to supply deltoid, teres minor and a small patch of skin over the upper lateral part of the humerus. It is most frequently damaged in shoulder dislocations, and must be tested **before** relocation to make sure that any damage is not unfairly attributed to the doctor!

3 – a

The radial nerve appears in the lateral part of the antecubital fossa under brachioradialis, and divides into a superficial branch and deep branch. The superficial branch is sensory only, whereas the deep branch supplies all of the finger and wrist extensors that are found in the posterior compartment of the forearm.

Question 6:
Theme: Fracture management

Options:

- a Cast splint (Plaster of Paris)
- b Open reduction and internal fixation
- c Open reduction with external fixation
- d Traction
- e Functional bracing
- f Conservative (protection alone)

For each of the fractures described below, select the single most likely method of treatment from the options listed above. Each option may be used once, more than once or not at all.

1. A 19-year-old factory worker traps his right leg in an industrial machine. He sustains an open fracture of his right tibia and fibula. The surrounding soft tissue is badly macerated.

2. A 41-year-old woman everts her left foot while running. Her ankle becomes tender and swollen and she can not weight bear on that side. X-ray reveals a minimally displaced fracture of the lateral malleolus below the inferior tibiofibular joint.

3. A 25-year-old man falls off his motorbike at 40 mph. X-ray reveals that he has suffered a supracondylar fracture of his left femur, which is initially treated for 6 weeks on traction after successful closed reduction.

Question 6: Answers

1 – c
External fixation is particularly useful for fractures with severe soft tissue damage.

2 – a
There is no need for an open reduction here – the ankle joint is stable as the fracture has occurred **beneath** the inferior tibio-fibular joint.

Ankle fractures are commonly categorized using the Weber classification:

- **A** = fracture is below the distal tibio-fibular joint (a syndesmosis)
- **B** = fracture is at the level of the level of the syndesmosis
- **C** = fracture is above the level of the syndesmosis

Weber B and C fractures inherently produce an unstable ankle joint, and are therefore likely to need open reduction and fixation.

3 – e
A functional cast/brace is a form of external splinting of a fracture. It is most often used 3–6 weeks after femoral or tibial fractures when the complete leg cast is removed. A plaster (or another material) is then applied to the limb above and below the knee joint, and these are connected by a hinge that goes across the joint. This allows the knee joint to be mobilised while still holding the fracture in position. It is therefore helpful in reducing joint stiffness.

Treatment	Advantages	Disadvantages
Plaster of Paris	Safe and the reduced fracture is held in position	Patient unable to move the joint, which may then become stiff
Traction	Safe	Patient stays in hospital a long time. Cannot hold fracture, although may keep length
Operative fixation	Early. Patient may be able to move the joint. Fracture is held in position	Safety is a concern due to complications of surgery

Question 7:
Theme: Complications of fractures

Options:
- a Sudek's atrophy (algodystrophy)
- b Compartment syndrome
- c Non-union
- d Osteoarthritis
- e Vascular injury
- f Malunion
- g Haemorrhage
- h Avascular necrosis

For each of the situations described below, select the single most likely complication from the options listed above. Each option may be used once, more than once or not at all.

1. A 21-year-old woman suffers a closed fracture of her left tibia and fibula after falling over while skiing off piste. At hospital it is noted that her pain is even greater than would be expected for such an injury, especially on passive toe extension. The ankle pulses are present, and there is no neurological loss.

2. A 26-year-old window cleaner falls off his ladder onto his outstretched left hand. He fractures his scaphoid bone, which is treated with a scaphoid plaster and appears to be healing well. He re-presents due to development of a burning feeling in his left hand with accompanying swelling and erythema.

3. A 73-year-old woman falls and fractures the mid-shaft of her left humerus. There is no distal neurovascular deficit. Three months after injury she can angulate her distal humerus on her proximal humerus with no pain.

Question 7: Answers

1 – b
An increase in pressure in a fascial compartment may occur either by bleeding from a vessel, or simply by post-traumatic oedema. Eventually this will lead to venous and finally arterial obstruction with resulting ischaemia. It is not possible for the muscle to regenerate; instead dead muscle is replaced by fibrous tissue, which results in contractures (Volkmann's ischaemic contracture). Pain is the presenting feature: it is important to realise that a pulse will still be present until the later stages of this process. A simple clinical test is pain on passive stretching of the compartment. It is treated by prompt fasciotomy.

2 – a
Algodystrophy is a poorly understood condition that may occur after any injury; its preferred name is **reflex sympathetic dystrophy**. It is believed to be due to an abnormality in the sympathetic nervous system in which the area concerned feels hot and swollen at first, and subsequently the skin becomes pale and atrophic. A burning pain accompanies it, and an X-ray of the affected area may show patches of osteoporosis. At the wrist the condition is known as Sudek's atrophy.

Treatment is largely by physiotherapy and analgesics. The use of the surgical sympathetic block is now under debate, and medical treatment with carbamazepine or amitryptiline is becoming more common.

3 – c
Non-union of a fracture is exactly that: the fracture does not heal, and it is possible painlessly to move the distal and proximal fragments on each other. The ends may either be smooth and sclerotic (atrophic non-union), or they may be active and ragged (hypertrophic non-union).

Non-union is likely to occur if a delayed union is left untreated, or if the fracture ends are separated. This may occur if muscle or cartilage is interposed, or if the ends are pulled apart by muscle.

Malunion of a fracture is said to occur when the bones join in an unsatisfactory position.

Question 8:
Theme: Spinal injuries

Options:

      a Jefferson fracture
      b Hangman's fracture
      c Cord transection at C6 level
      d Spinal shock
      e Brown–Sequard syndrome
      f Cauda equina syndrome

For each of the signs below, select the single most likely diagnosis from the options listed above. Each option may be used once, more than once, or not at all.

1. A 15-year-old boy dives into a shallow swimming pool and hits his head on the bottom. There is distension of the abdomen with inspiration.

2. A 56-year-old vet crashes his car into a cow. His head hits the windscreen, hyperextending his neck. There is a fracture of the pedicle of C2 on his radiograph.

3. A 33-year-old scaffolder falls 5 metres onto his back. He is rendered paraplegic, has decreased tone, areflexia and complete anaesthesia in his lower limbs. He has retention of urine lasting 3 weeks, at which time he becomes hyper-reflexic.

Question 8: Answers

1 – c

The phrenic nerve is motor and sensory to the diaphragm. Remember that 'C3,4,5 keeps the diaphragm alive'. Therefore, a lesion below C5 will not affect diaphragmatic function, but **will** paralyse all intercostal muscles below the level of section. Breathing will therefore be totally reliant on the diaphragm and the muscles of the neck, resulting in a far more obvious diaphragmatic movement on inspiration.

2 – b

This is the classic presentation of a Hangman's fracture. As it is caused by distraction (a pull from hyperextension), do not treat with traction but rather with immobilization in a halo-body cast for 12 weeks.

3 – d

Spinal shock occurs after severe spinal cord injury. There is dysfunction to the cord below the injury, which causes areflexic flaccid paralysis. This may last from 3 days to 8 weeks, the average being 3–4 weeks, which is heralded by minimal reflex activity.

Cauda equina syndrome affects nerve roots and therefore has dermatomal signs. It affects lower levels than spinal shock.

A Jefferson fracture is due to a direct blow to the top of the head. This causes the ring of the atlas to shatter – as if one had trodden on a polo mint.

Question 9:
Theme: Tendon anatomy and injury

Options:
- a Tibialis anterior
- b Extensor indicis
- c Flexor digitorum profundus (FDP)
- d Flexor digitorum superficialis (FDS)
- e Flexor carpi ulnaris
- f Peroneus brevis
- g Peroneus longus
- h Extensor hallucis longus
- i Extensor digitorum longus

For each of the descriptions below, select the single most likely tendon involved from the options listed above. Each option may be used once, more than once or not at all.

1. A 32-year-old man violently inverts his right ankle while playing football. X-ray reveals that he has fractured the base of his right fifth metatarsal.

2. A 26-year-old chef cut his left index finger while trying to open an oyster. On examination he has a cut on the volar aspect of his left index finger, and can not flex the finger at the proximal interphalangeal (IP) joint with the distal IP joint kept in extension. Flexion at the distal interphalangeal joint is preserved.

3. The dorsalis pedis pulse is felt lateral to this tendon.

Question 9: Answers

1 – f

Peroneus brevis arises from the lateral side of the fibula. Its tendon winds around the posterior aspect of the lateral malleolus and inserts into the styloid process (base) of the fifth metatarsal. Violent and sudden ankle inversion may therefore cause an avulsion injury of the base of the fifth metatarsal, as has happened to the man in this case. (Note that peroneus tertius also inserts on the fifth metatarsal's styloid process.)

2 – d

There are two muscles that flex the finger: flexor digitorum profundus (FDP) and flexor digitorum superficialis (FDS).

This man has divided the FDS tendon to his left index finger. FDP attaches to the distal phalanx and can be tested by seeing if the patient can flex the distal interphalangeal (DIP) joint with the proximal inter-phalangeal (PIP) joint held in full extension.

FDS attaches to the middle phalanx and can be tested by seeing if the patient can flex his PIP joint with his DIP joint fully extended.

3 – h

The dorsalis pedis artery is the continuation of the anterior tibial artery, which is a branch of the popliteal artery. It can be felt on the dorsum of the foot between the tendons of extensor hallucis longus (medially) and extensor digitorum longus (laterally). The tendon of tibialis anterior is **medial** to the tendon of extensor hallucis longus – you can feel these on yourself.

Question 10:
Theme: Burns

Options:

a   810 ml
b   1080 ml
c   4050 ml
d   4860 ml
e   5400 ml
f   6480 ml
g   7200 ml

For each of the clinical scenarios below, using the Muir–Barclay formula, select the single most likely volume of fluid replacement that should be given over the first day from the options listed above. Each option may be used once, more than once, or not at all.

1. A 29-year-old man is rescued from a house fire. He has full-thickness burns covering the entire front of his chest and the anterior aspects of both arms and forearms. His face and genitalia have been spared. His weight is 80 kg.

2. An 81-year-old woman spills a pan of boiling milk over herself. She sustains full-thickness burns to the whole of her left arm and left leg. She weighs 60 kg.

Question 10: Answers

1 – e

[(4.5 + 4.5 + 18 × 80)]/2 = 1080 ml for first 4 h. Total in 24 h = **5400 ml** (see below for fluid regimen)

2 – c

[(9 + 18) × 60]/2 = 810 ml for first 4 h. Total in 24 h = **4050 ml** (see below for fluid regimen)

The main worry with burns is plasma loss and therefore hypovolaemia, which can be deceptively large. Several formulae have been adopted to calculate the fluid regimen that patients must receive to correct this loss. We have used the Muir–Barclay formula, which is well known.

First, it is necessary to weigh the patient. The surface area of the burn must then be calculated. This may be estimated using the 'rule of nines'.

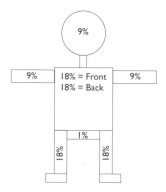

- In a 1-year-old child the head and neck = 18% surface area
- In a 5-year-old child the head and neck = 13% surface area
- Adult neck = 1% surface area
- Patient's hand = 1% of their surface area (useful to assess patchy areas of burn)

The amount of fluid per unit time is now calculated using the **Muir–Barclay formula**:

[% surface area burn × mass (kg)]/2 = volume of fluid (ml)

This volume of fluid is then given intravenously:

- every 4 h for 12 h (i.e. 3 units of time), then
- every 6 h for 12 h (i.e. 2 units of time), then
- once over 12 h (i.e. 1 unit of time).

It is important continuously to reassess the patient during this time.

Core Module 4: Intensive Care

Questions

1	Chest conditions	69
2	Complications of central venous cannulation	71
3	Shock	73
4	Anatomy of the diaphragm	75
5	Lung volumes	77
6	Respiratory failure	79
7	Applied anatomy of the great vessels	81
8	Metabolic abnormalities	83
9	Ward allocation	85
10	Anatomy of the thorax	87

Question 1:
Theme: Chest conditions

Options:

a   Massive haemothorax
b   Tension pneumothorax
c   Cardiac tamponade
d   Aortic dissection
e   Superior vena cava obstruction

For each of the physical signs described below, select the single most likely diagnosis from the options listed above. Each option may be used once, more than once, or not at all.

1.   Fixed, raised JVP.

2.   Rising JVP on inspiration with normal breath sounds.

Question 1: Answers

1 – e

Obstruction of the superior vena cava (SVC) will result in a **fixed**, raised JVP. Causes of an SVC obstruction are:

- Carcinoma of the lung (primary and/or lymph nodes)
- Lymphoma
- Aortic aneurysm
- Mediastinal goitre
- Mediastinal fibrosis

2 – c

Inspiration decreases the intrathoracic pressure, sucking the contents of the venous system into the right atrium and causing the JVP to fall. A cardiac tamponade acts as a constrictive band around the heart. As less blood can now enter the right atrium, a rise in JVP will be seen on inspiration.

Question 2:
Theme: Complications of central venous cannulation

Options:

    a   Tension pneumothorax
    b   Arterial puncture
    c   Massive chylothorax
    d   Air embolism
    e   Infection of cannulation site
    f   Catheter misplacement
    g   Embolisation of broken catheter tip

For each of the complications described below, select the single most likely cause from the options listed above. Each option may be used once, more than once, or not at all.

1. Twenty minutes after attempted insertion of a central line into the right subclavian vein of a 74-year-old man, he becomes unresponsive. On examination he is pale, tachycardic and profoundly hypotensive. He has dullness to percussion on the right side of his chest with reduced breath sounds. His central venous pressure is low.

2. Two days after insertion of a central line, a patient complains of localised pleuritic chest pain. On examination his respiratory rate is 18 breaths min^{-1}. Chest auscultation reveals a pleural rub over the painful area. Chest X-ray shows a radio opaque density at the left hilum.

Question 2: Answers

1 – b
This patient has suffered a large haemorrhage after puncture of his right subclavian artery, which has bled into his thoracic cavity. Hence, he has the signs and symptoms of a massive haemothorax.

2 – g
The catheter tip has broken off and has embolised to the lung, producing the features of pulmonary infarction.

This should not be confused with an air embolism, which has three common causes:

- After insertion of the line in a supine patient, a port is left open. This lies above the level of the heart if the patient is sat upright. Air becomes introduced into the system and shock rapidly develops
- When the line is removed, a track remains from the skin to the underlying vein. Air may enter this track, also producing a rapid shock
- Air is inadvertently introduced into the line by mistake, e.g. while trying to pass air into a nasogastric tube

Question 3:
Theme: Shock

Options:

a   Septic shock
b   Cardiogenic shock
c   Hypovolaemic shock
d   Anaphylactic shock
e   Neurogenic shock
f   Electric shock

For each of the cases described below, select the single most likely cause from the options listed above. Each option may be used once, more than once, or not at all.

1. A 67-year-old man is recovering in the Intensive Care Unit after repair of a perforated colonic diverticulum. He becomes rapidly unwell, with a heart rate $= 150$ beats min^{-1} and a BP $= 90/50$ mmHg. His peripheries are warm and his JVP is reduced.

2. A 26-year-old woman falls off her motorbike at 40 mph. She has a heart rate $= 50$ beats min^{-1} and a blood pressure $= 83/46$ mmHg. She has warm peripheries and a low JVP.

3. Odd one out.

Question 3: Answers

1 – a
Septic shock is likely to occur as a result of **endo**toxins produced by Gram-negative bacteria. These cause both vasodilatation and leaky capillary walls, resulting in hypotension. Cells damaged by endotoxins release proteolytic enzymes, which causes further leakage by paralysing precapillary sphincters. The endotoxin also acts as a negative inotrope.

2 – e
Damage to the spinal cord may stop sympathetic function below the level of the injury. The resulting vasodilatation may then produce hypovolaemia with warm peripheries. Moreover, the heart may be affected depending on whether the lesion is **below** or **above** the level of T6.

- An injury above T6 will diminish the sympathetic outflow to the heart. A profound bradycardia will therefore be seen instead. The heart will also not respond to hypovolaemia with the expected reflex tachycardia. Any stimulation of the parasympathetic system via the vagus nerve will worsen the bradycardia and may cause cardiac arrest. This can be achieved simply by pharyngeal suction.
- An injury below T6 will spare the heart, and the shock will be recognised by its effect on bladder function with warm peripheries.

3 – f
Surgical humour (ho ho ho).

Shock	HR	BP	CVP	CO	Periphery	Treatment
Hypovolaemic	↑	↓	↓	↓	Cool	Fluids
Anaphylactic	↑	↓	↓	↓	Warm	Adrenaline
Septic	↑	↓	↓	↑	Warm	Vasoconstrictors/ antibiotics
Cardiogenic	↑	↓	↑	↓	Cool	Inotropes
Neurogenic	↑ or ↓	↓	↓	↑ or ↓	Warm	Fluids/ vasopressors

HR, heart rate; BP, blood pressure; CVP, central venous pressure; CO, cardiac output

Question 4:
Theme: Anatomy of the diaphragm

Options:

      a   Aortic opening (T12)
      b   Oesophageal opening (T10)
      c   Inferior vena caval opening (T8)
      d   None of the above

For each of the structures described below, select the diaphragmatic opening through which it passes from the options listed above. Each option may be used once, more than once, or not at all.

1. Azygos vein.

2. Left vagus nerve.

3. Left phrenic nerve.

4. Right phrenic nerve.

Question 4: Answers

1 – a

2 – b

3 – d

4 – c

Through the <u>aortic opening</u> (median arcuate ligament) formed by the left and right crus (T12):

- Aorta
- Azygos vein
- Thoracic duct

Through the <u>oesophageal opening</u> through a loop of the right crus (T10):

- Oesophagus
- Left and right vagi
- Left gastric artery and vein

Through the <u>caval opening</u> in the central tendon (T8):

- Inferior vena cava
- Right phrenic nerve

The left phrenic nerve dives directly into the diaphragm's central tendon and therefore does not pass through any of the openings above.

The left and right sympathetic chains pass either side of the aorta, but do not pass through the aortic opening itself. They pass underneath the **medial arcuate ligament**, which is formed by a thickening of the fascia of psoas that stretches between the lower L1 vertebral body (or L2) to the transverse process of L1 at the lateral margin of psoas.

The **lateral arcuate ligament**, which is a thickening of the lumbar fascia, extends from the L1 transverse process to the twelfth rib, where it is in contact with the lateral border of quadratus lumborum. The subcostal nerve and vessels pass through it on each side.

The splanchnic nerves pierce their ipsilateral crus.

The superior epigastric vessels pass between the xiphisternum and costal fibres of the diaphragm.

Question 5:
Theme: Lung volumes

Options:

a   Residual volume (RV)
b   Total lung capacity (TLC)
c   Functional residual capacity (FRC)
d   Vital capacity (VC)
e   Inspiratory reserve volume (IRV)
f   Expiratory reserve volume (ERV)
g   Tidal volume (TV)

For each of the equations described below, select the answer from the options listed above. Each option may be used once, more than once, or not at all.

1. $TLC - VC = ?$

2. $RV + ERV = ?$

3. $VC - (IRV + ERV) = ?$

Question 5: Answers

1 – a
TLC – VC = RV

2 – c
RV + ERV = FRC

3 – g
VC – (IRV + ERV) = TV

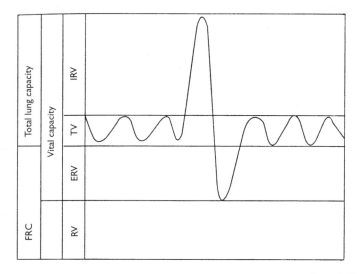

Basic spirometry. RV = Residual volume; ERV = expiratory reserve volume; TV = tidal volume; IRV = inspiratory reserve volume; FRC = functional residual capacity.

Question 6:
Theme: Respiratory failure

Options:

      a O_2, antibiotics and physiotherapy
      b O_2 and anticoagulation
      c O_2, aspiration and drainage
      d O_2, morphine, diuretics and nitrates
      e O_2, airway control and surgery

For each of the clinical vignettes described below, select the single most likely management from the options listed above. Each option may be used once, more than once, or not at all.

1. A 67-year-old man wakes up breathless in the middle of the night, coughing up frothy sputum. He has a history of ischaemic heart disease. On examination he is apyrexial and there are coarse inspiratory crackles in both lung bases.

2. A 65-year-old woman is undergoing palliative treatment for her left-sided breast carcinoma. She becomes progressively breathless over 1 week. On examination her respiratory rate = 32 breaths min^{-1}. She has decreased chest expansion on her left side, with stony dullness to percussion up to the left fourth rib. There are no breath sounds over this area.

3. A 74-year-old woman presents to the Accident and Emergency Department with shortness of breath. She had noticed an enlarging neck lump over the past 3 months. On examination there is a large goitre. She has marked inspiratory stridor, and her oxygen saturation is 82% on air.

Question 6: Answers

1 – d

This man has pulmonary oedema. Diuretics and morphine decrease pre-load, and nitrates decrease afterload.

2 – c

This woman has a pleural effusion. Do not let her return home without draining it.

3 – e

It is vital to secure an airway in this patient with subglottic stenosis.

Question 7:
Theme: Applied anatomy of the great vessels

Options:

    a   Aortic dissection
    b   Cervical rib
    c   Subclavian steal syndrome
    d   Takayasu's arteritis
    e   Patent ductus arteriosus
    f   Coarctation of the aorta

For each of the case scenarios described below, select the single most likely diagnosis from the options listed above. Each option may be used once, more than once, or not at all.

1. A 45-year-old man notices that he feels dizzy when he plays tennis, with a cramping pain in his left arm. While pumping up his bicycle tyre one day he passes out and is taken to hospital.

2. A 23-year-old Asian woman feels unwell and suffers dizziness, especially on turning her head. On examination blood pressure = 170/120. Despite being well hydrated, no pulses can be felt in the extremities. She has a systolic heart murmur.

3. A 24-year-old man is noticed to have rib notching on his chest X-ray during routine army medical examination. He has a systolic murmur, loudest at the fourth intercostal space posteriorly.

Question 7: Answers

1 – c
Subclavian steal syndrome occurs when there is a blockage in the first part of the subclavian artery **proximal** to the origin of the vertebral artery. If the arm is used then blood will reach it by reverse flow down the vertebral artery (subclavian 'steal'). The subsequent lack of blood flow to the brain may render the patient dizzy or even unconscious. It can be easily corrected with a bypass graft, usually between the subclavian and the common carotid artery.

In contrast, a cervical rib may press on the subclavian artery causing thoracic outlet syndrome. It may also compress the C8 and T1 nerve roots, resulting in wasting of the small muscles of the hand and the corresponding anaesthesia.

2 – d
Takayasu's arteritis is very rare and typically affects young Asian women. It is an arteritis of the aorta, the first few centimetres of the carotid and brachiocephalic trunk and/or renal arteries (which causes hypertension). Ophthalmic symptoms vary as do CNS symptoms (from dizziness to hemiplegia and fits). The classic description will always mention **pulselessness** in the peripheries, but note that the systolic murmurs are above and below the clavicles.

3 – f
Coarctation of the aorta usually occurs where the remnant of the ductus arteriosus acts as a constrictive band around the aorta, i.e. just **distal** to the left subclavian artery origin. Patients may have dyspnoea on exertion and/or cerebrovascular accidents. On examination there is radio-femoral delay (and weak left arm pulses in the 2% who have coarctation **proximal** to the left subclavian artery).

Collateral blood vessels develop to try and provide blood distal to the block. More blood flows down the internal thoracic (mammary) artery into the intercostals. Some will flow into the aorta, and some will continue into the superior and then inferior epigastric arteries to supply the lower limb.

A CXR will show rib notching due to enlarged intercostal arteries.

Question 8:
Theme: Metabolic abnormalities

Options:

a Hypokalaemia
b Hyperkalaemia
c Hyperglycaemia
d Hypophosphataemia
e Hyperphosphataemia

For each of the patients described below, select the single most likely metabolic abnormality from the options listed above. Each option may be used once, more than once, or not at all.

1. A 52-year-old alcoholic receives a feeding jejunostomy 3 days after rupturing his oesophagus while vomiting. Feeding is now introduced.

2. A 25-year-old man presents having suffered an electric shock. He is systemically well and appears to be recovering well despite a partial thickness burn to his right arm. He develops proteinuria, and his serum creatine kinase becomes elevated.

3. A 61-year-old woman with heart failure is started on oral prednisolone for an exacerbation of her chronic obstructive pulmonary disease. She regularly takes oral frusemide.

Question 8: Answers

1 – d

Hypophosphataemia occurs during acute alcohol withdrawal. It is also a risk when giving carbohydrate after fasting, e.g. total parenteral nutrition or anorexia nervosa.

2 – b

Electric shock releases myoglobin from the damaged muscle cells, i.e. rhabdomyolysis. This blocks the renal tubules causing acute renal failure and consequent hyperkalaemia.

3 – a

Both loop diuretics and corticosteroids cause hypokalaemia.

Question 9:
Theme: Ward allocation

Options:

     a   Intensive care unit (ICU)
     b   High-dependency unit (HDU)
     c   Surgical ward
     d   Discharge

For each of the clinical vignettes described below, select the single most likely destination from the options listed above. Each option may be used once, more than once, or not at all.

1. A 70-year-old man undergoes an elective aortic valve replacement.

2. A 72-year-old woman fractures the neck of her right femur. She has insulin-dependent diabetes mellitus, has suffered a myocardial infarction in the past and is on warfarin for a recent DVT.

3. A 26-year-old van driver is thrown through his windscreen in a road traffic accident. He has a flail chest for which he is intubated and ventilated.

Question 9: Answers

1 – a

2 – b

3 – a

The ICU is an area for treatment of patients with, or at high risk of developing, organ failure. This includes patients on mechanical ventilation.

The HDU is an appropriate area for patients needing monitoring and nursing input above that which a general ward can offer.

Question 10:
Theme: Anatomy of the thorax

Options:

- a Azygos vein
- b Hemi-azygos vein
- c Inferior vena cava
- d Thoracic duct
- e Parietal pleura
- f Visceral pleura

For each of the descriptions below, select the single most likely structure from the options listed above. Each option may be used once, more than once, or not at all.

1. This structure enters the venous system at the junction of the left subclavian and left internal jugular veins.

2. This structure enters the venous system at the superior vena cava.

3. The sensation of this structure is supplied by the somatic nervous system.

Question 10: Answers

1 – d

The thoracic duct originates from the cisterna chyli under the diaphragm, to the right of the aorta. It passes posterior to the diaphragm with the aorta, and ascends in the thorax behind the oesophagus until it reaches T5, where it crosses the midline and continues upwards. It then runs behind the carotid sheath and hooks over the subclavian artery to drain into the junction formed by the left subclavian vein (laterally) and the internal jugular vein (medially).

The thoracic duct drains all of the lymphatics below the diaphragm, as well as the left side of the thorax, left head and neck and left upper limb. It may be damaged by the insertion of a central venous line into the left subclavian vein, causing a chylothorax.

2 – a

The azygos vein is formed by the ascending lumbar veins and the lower 11 intercostal veins on the right side of the thorax. It lies medial to the sympathetic trunk and is joined at the T4 level by the hemi-azygos vein, which drains the left side of the thorax. It arches over the root of the right lung and terminates by draining into the superior vena cava.

3 – e

The sensation of the pleura is as follows:

- The visceral pleura is innervated by the autonomic nervous system, and is therefore sensitive to stretch but not to pain and touch.
- The parietal pleura is innervated by the somatic nervous system and is therefore sensitive to pain and touch. The parietal pleura is supplied thus:
  - Costal pleura – intercostal nerves
  - Mediastinal and **central** diaphragmatic pleura – phrenic nerve
  - **Peripheral** diaphragmatic pleura – lower five or six intercostal nerves

Pleuritic chest pain will arise as a result of inflammation of the **parietal** pleura.

Note the important T4 level, where you will find:

- Manubriosternal joint (angle of Louis)
- Second costal cartilage (and second rib)
- Base of the arch of the aorta (goes up to T2 and then back down again)
- Carina
- Crossing of the hemi-azygos vein to join to azygos vein
- Crossing of the thoracic duct from right to left (T5 also)
- Ligamentum arteriosum
- The division between the superior and inferior mediastinum

Core Module 5: Neoplasia

Questions

1	Colorectal cancer	91
2	Tumour markers	93
3	Cytotoxic chemotherapy	95
4	Skin lesions	97
5	Breast lumps	99
6	Breast cancer	101
7	Oncogenes	103
8	Thyroid neoplasia	105
9	Lung cancer	107
10	Care of the terminally ill patient	109

Question 1:
Theme: Colorectal cancer

Options:

    a   Left hemicolectomy
    b   Right hemicolectomy
    c   Sigmoid colectomy
    d   Anterior resection
    e   Abdomino-perineal resection
    f   Hartmann's procedure
    g   Anterior resection + intravenous 5-FU

For each of the patients described below, select the single most likely treatment from the options listed above. Each option may be used once, more than once or not at all.

1. A 61-year-old man is discovered at sigmoidoscopy to have a rectal tumour that is 2 cm from the anal verge.

2. A 60-year-old woman presents with a change in bowel habit. Sigmoidoscopy and biopsy demonstrates a rectal tumour 10 cm from the anal verge. Ultrasound reveals multiple metastases in the left lobe of the liver.

Question 1: Answers

1 – e

2 – g

The anatomical blood supply and the accessibility of the tumour guide surgery for resection of colorectal carcinoma.

The **foregut** is supplied by the coeliac axis. This supplies bowel from the distal oesophagus to the second part of the duodenum.

The **superior mesenteric artery supplies the midgut**. This supplies bowel from the second part of the duodenum to two-thirds of the way across the transverse colon.

The **inferior mesenteric artery supplies the hindgut**. This supplies the bowel from two-thirds of the way across the transverse colon to the mid-rectum.

Below 5 cm from the anal verge there will not be enough bowel left for an anastomosis to be formed. In these cases an abdomino-perineal resection is performed with permanent colostomy.

In acute obstruction and/or the patient is unwell one may perform a Hartmann's operation instead, as it is quick, clean and safe.

One may consider resection of liver metastases if there are three or less confined to one lobe, with no other disease and a 2 cm margin. If there are multiple metastases, one can administer palliative chemotherapy. Currently, administration of 5-FU via the portal vein prolongs life expectancy. It is thought to kill cells showered into the bloodstream when the tumour is handled peri-operatively.

Question 2:
Theme: Tumour markers

Options:

     a CA-125
     b PSA
     c CEA
     d α-FP
     e LDH

For each of the neoplasms described below, select the single most likely tumour marker from the options listed above. Each option may be used once, more than once or not at all.

1. Ovarian carcinoma.

2. Testicular teratoma.

3. Testicular seminoma.

4. Hepatocellular carcinoma.

Question 2: Answers

1 – a

2 – d

3 – e

4 – d

Tumour	Tumour marker
Ovarian carcinoma	CA-125
Testicular teratoma	β-HCG, α-FP
Testicular seminoma	β-HCG, LDH
Hepatocellular carcinoma	α-FP
Prostatic carcinoma	PSA
Colorectal carcinoma	CEA

Question 3:
Theme: Cytotoxic chemotherapy

Options:

      a   Methotrexate
      b   Mitomycin C
      c   Vincristine
      d   Cisplatin
      e   Paclitaxel
      f   None of the above

For each of the medications listed below, select the single most likely chemotherapeutic agent from the options listed above. Each option may be used once, more than once or not at all.

1. This drug is an antimetabolite.

2. This drug is an anti-tumour antibiotic.

3. This drug is an alkylating agent.

Question 3: Answers

1 – a

2 – b

3 – d

Class	Mechanism	Drugs
Alkylating agents	Binds to DNA, impeding replication	Cisplatin, cyclophosphamide, chlorambucil, melphalan
Antimetabolites	Impede DNA synthesis	Methotrexate, 5–fluorouracil, 6–mercaptopurine
Vinca alkaloids	Prevent formation of mitotic spindle	Vincristine, vinblastine, vindesine, etoposide
Anti-tumour antibiotics	Varies between antibiotics	Bleomycin, doxyrubicin, mitomycin C

Question 4:
Theme: Skin lesions

Options:
- a   Basal cell carcinoma
- b   Squamous cell carcinoma
- c   Malignant melanoma
- d   Keratoacanthoma
- e   Kaposi's sarcoma
- f   Junctional naevus
- g   Strawberry naevus
- h   Blue naevus

For each of the cases described below, select the single most likely skin lesion from the options listed above. Each option may be used once, more than once or not at all.

1. A 56-year-old man presents with multiple hard lumps in his right groin. Examination reveals a discoloured lesion under the nail of his right hallux which is distorting the nail.

2. A 33-year-old woman presents with a 7 mm dark brown lesion just below the lateral malleolus of her left ankle. There is a similar 2 mm lesion directly adjacent to it. Neither lesions were present on her last summer holiday and they both bleed on contact.

3. Current guidelines advise that this lesion is resected with a 5 mm margin.

Question 4: Answers

1 – c

2 – c

There are five types of malignant melanoma of the skin:

- **Superficial spreading** – most common; usually palpable; irregular edge
- **Lentigo maligna** – least common; least malignant; usually on the face of the elderly (also known as Hutchinson's freckle)
- **Nodular** – most malignant; affects the young; may ulcerate and bleed
- **Acral** – affects palms and soles (includes subungal tumours); poor prognosis
- **Amelanotic** – pink, but usually pigmented at base; terrible prognosis

You may be asked to see a patient with **one yellow eye**. This is a spot diagnosis – can you guess what it is? To work it out:

- Why is only one eye yellow? Jaundice should be seen in both eyes; therefore one eye must be false
- Why is the patient jaundiced? There is liver pathology (in this case)
- How are the above connected? The patient has had a malignant melanoma of the eye which was removed, but there is late spread to the liver

Malignant melanoma of the eye originates from the pigment cells of the choroid or the iris. Liver secondaries can occur 20 years after the tumour is removed.

3 – a

Resection margins for different skin tumours are as follows:

- Basal cell carcinoma – 5 mm (if not cured by radiotherapy first)
- Squamous cell carcinoma – 1 cm
- Malignant melanoma – depends on stage, e.g. Breslow staging (as below):

Depth of lesion (mm)	Recommended width of excision (mm)
< 0.75	2 (i.e. biopsy)
0.76–1.5	20
1.6–3.0	50
> 3.0	50

Source: *Bailey and Love's Short Practice of Surgery* (Berlin: Springer)

Question 5:
Theme: Breast lumps

Options:

- a   Fibroadenoma
- b   Duct papilloma
- c   Duct ectasia
- d   Fibrocystic disease
- e   Fat necrosis
- f   Phylloides tumour
- g   Paget's disease

For each of the clinical vignettes listed below, select the single most likely diagnosis from the options listed above. Each option may be used once, more than once or not at all.

1. A 48-year-old air hostess presents with a creamy green discharge that is sometimes bloodstained from her left nipple. She has subsequently developed a tender lump in her left breast. On examination, a 1 cm firm mass is palpated just under the areola of her breast with surrounding erythema.

2. A 40-year-old radiographer presents with a dark bloody discharge from her right breast. On examination there is a firm mass under her areola, and when pressed blood escapes from the nipple.

3. A 24-year-old doctor presents with a non-tender lump in her right breast. It is 2 cm in diameter, hard and well circumscribed. When testing for fluctuance it slips easily between the fingers.

Question 5: Answers

1 – c

Duct ectasia usually occurs around the age of the menopause. It is thought that hypertrophy of the duct epithelium causes duct blockage, with resultant proximal dilatation (ectasia). It classically produces a creamy green discharge with the consistency of toothpaste. It may be confused with breast cancer due to the presence of a lump, especially if it forms an abscess (causing periductal mastitis) which may retract the nipple.

2 – b

A papilloma within the duct tends to bleed. If there is bloody discharge from a nipple, one must always exclude carcinoma. Beware of multiple papillomas (rare), which are **premalignant**.

3 – a

The mobile nature if a fibroadenoma has given it the nickname 'breast mouse'. It typically presents in younger women (18–25 years) and has a very small (1:1000) risk of malignancy. It does not require resection if small and FNAC is normal; most are excised for reassurance and histological confirmation.

Question 6:
Theme: Breast cancer

Options:

a   Wide local excision
b   Wide local excision + breast radiotherapy
c   Wide local excision + breast radiotherapy + axillary clearance
d   Mastectomy
e   Mastectomy + axillary clearance
f   Tamoxifen
g   Cytotoxic chemotherapy
h   Tamoxifen + cytotoxic chemotherapy
i   Bilateral oophorectomy
j   Local radiotherapy

For each of the case scenarios listed below, select the single most likely therapy from the options listed above. Each option may be used once, more than once or not at all.

1. Investigation of a 35-year-old woman with an inverted nipple reveals a carcinoma of her right breast with no palpable axillary lymph nodes. She has expressed concern regarding disfiguring surgery.

2. A 50-year-old postmenopausal woman undergoes a simple mastectomy with lymph node sampling following a diagnosis of breast carcinoma. Histology reveals carcinoma in three of the four sampled nodes. The tumour is oestrogen receptor negative.

Question 6: Answers

1 – c

2 – h

There is still much debate over a definitive treatment regime for breast cancer. In general:

Assessment: 'Triple assessment'

        a) Clinical

        b) Radiological (ultrasound/mammogram)

        c) Pathological (FNAC)

Staging: via the UICC TNM classification (please refer to *Aird's*)

Treatment: (Source: *Improving Outcomes in Breast Cancer*. NHS executive)

1. The Breast

As *there appears to be no difference between surgical procedures in terms of overall survival*, the operation performed will be decided on an individual basis after discussion between the patient and consultant. Options are:

- Wide local excision (WLE) + radiotherapy to remaining breast
- Mastectomy ± immediate reconstruction **or** delayed reconstruction

2. The Axilla

Axillary lymph node status is the most powerful prognostic indicator for breast cancer. Thus in **all** patients the axilla should be staged by sampling at least four nodes, or by clearance. The choice between sampling and clearance is controversial, and made on an individual patient basis.

Radiotherapy to the axilla may be omitted if there is a negative sample of at least four nodes. There is normally no need for radiotherapy to the axilla if axillary **clearance**, rather than axillary sampling, is performed.

3. Adjuvant therapy

The prognosis of breast cancer is affected by the presence of 'micro-metastases'.

- **Tamoxifen** – usually given to **all** groups of patients, including those with recurrent disease, greatest effects when primary tumour is oestrogen receptor +ve
- **Ovarian ablation** – same effectiveness as chemotherapy for pre-menopausal women
- **Chemotherapy** – more effective in younger women, though still useful in older women

Question 7:
Theme: Oncogenes

Options:

    a erb
    b myc
    c ras
    d p53
    e DCC
    f BRCA-1
    g APC

For each of the descriptions listed below, select the single most likely onco-gene from the options listed above. Each option may be used once, more than once or not at all.

1. This oncogene is the single most common genetic alteration in human neoplasms.

2. Screening for familial adenomatous polyposis looks for this onco-gene.

3. This gene is inactivated in most colonic carcinomas.

Question 7: Answers

1 – d

2 – g
The *FAP* gene is the same as the *APC* (adenomatous polyposis coli) gene. It is on chromosome 5q 21.

3 – e
DCC stands for 'deleted in colon cancer'.

Oncogenes are genes that regulate cell proliferation and are found in the normal genome. They are dominant (**proto-**oncogenes) or recessive (**tumour suppressor genes**). The dominant genes will cause an uncontrolled cell proliferation when mutated.

p53 is a tumour suppressor gene, i.e. it needs to be suppressed, mutated or absent for a tumour to form. This is because products of these genes slow down cell proliferation. It is on chromosome 17p.

There is homozygous loss of the *p53* gene in almost all types of cancer, including lung, breast and colon cancer – the three most common causes of cancer deaths in the UK.

- **Proto-oncogenes** – *ras, myc, abl, erb*
- **Tumour suppressor genes** – *p53, DCC, APC, Rb* (retinoblastoma), *BRCA-1* (breast cancer)

Question 8:
Theme: Thyroid neoplasia

Options:
- a   Papillary carcinoma
- b   Follicular carcinoma
- c   Medullary carcinoma
- d   Anaplastic carcinoma
- e   Lymphoma
- f   Follicular adenoma

For each of the patients described below, select the single most likely diagnosis from the options listed above. Each option may be used once, more than once or not at all.

1. A 68-year-old woman presents with a rapidly enlarging lump in the neck and difficulty in breathing. On examination she is cachectic with a thyroid lump with cervical lymphadenopathy.

2. A 15-year-old girl presents with a thyroid lump. She has two enlarged ipsilateral cervical lymph nodes. FNAC reveals malignant cells with vesicular 'Orphan-Annie' nuclei.

Question 8: Answers

1 – d

2 – a

There are four main types of thyroid cancer:

Tumour	Age (years)	Sex	Histology	Spread	Prognosis
Papillary	10–40	F (commonest thyroid cancer)	Follicular structure; Orphan–Annie nuclei	Regional lymph nodes	Good
Follicular	40–60	F	Multiple foci of tumour rarely seen	Bloodstream	Moderate
Anaplastic	50–60	F	Poorly differentiated	Early lymph, bloodstream and direct spread	Poor
Medullary	Any age	M = F	Tumour of C-cells. Amyloid between cells	Lymphatics. Calcitonin is a tumour marker	Variable: good unless spread via bloodstream

Thyroid lymphoma is a rare condition, either as a primary or secondary site. It may be associated with Hashimoto's thyroiditis.

Question 9:
Theme: Lung cancer

Options:

    a Squamous cell carcinoma
    b Adenocarcinoma
    c Small cell carcinoma
    d Large cell undiferrentiated carcinoma

For each of the descriptions listed below, select the single most likely carcinoma from the options listed above. Each option may be used once, more than once or not at all.

1. This cancer has the best prognosis.

2. This cancer is most associated with smoking.

3. This cancer is usually found in the periphery of the lung.

4. Chemotherapy is the treatment of choice for most patients presenting with this cancer.

Question 9: Answers

1 – a
There are four types of lung cancer (excepting metastases):

- Small cell carcinoma ('oat cell' carcinoma)
- Adenocarcinoma ('non-small cell' carcinoma)
- Squamous cell carcinoma ('non-small cell' carcinoma)
- Large cell undifferentiated carcinoma

Squamous cell carcinoma has the **best** prognosis, followed by large cell, adeno- and finally small cell carcinoma.

2 – a
It is interesting to note that smoking has classically been associated with squamous cell carcinoma. Squamous cell carcinomas may produce parathyroid hormone leading to hypercalcaemia. This is an example of a **paraneoplastic syndrome**, which is defined as a condition due to the indirect effects of malignancy.

3 – b
Adenocarcinomas are found in the periphery of the lungs and are associated with conditions causing pulmonary fibrosis, especially asbestosis.

4 – c
Small cell carcinomas are also named 'oat cell' carcinomas because of the appearance of their nuclei. They have an appalling prognosis, with survival rare beyond 2 years. As the disease is usually well advanced at presentation, chemotherapy is most frequently used in these patients. This contrasts with non-small cell tumours, where it is possible to resect the tumour in 10–15% of cases.

As with squamous cell carcinomas, small cell tumours may cause paraneoplastic syndromes by secreting ACTH or ADH.

Question 10:
Theme: Care of the terminally ill patient

Options:

    a   Radiotherapy
    b   Tricyclic antidepressants
    c   Dexamethasone
    d   Diamorphine
    e   Diclofenac sodium
    f   Haloperidol
    g   Metoclopramide

For each of the clinical scenarios described below, select the single most likely treatment from the options listed above. Each option may be used once, more than once or not at all.

1. A 71-year-old woman presents with a personality change, confusion and drowsiness. She is known to be suffering from incurable carcinoma of the lung. A CT scan confirms multiple metastases in her brain.

2. A 69-year-old man is admitted for palliative treatment of his unresectable colonic carcinoma. He suffers severe nausea and vomiting from his opiate therapy.

3. A 83-year-old arthritic patient complains of back pain. Examination confirms that the pain is of bony origin.

Question 10: Answers

1 – c

Steroids are useful in decreasing raised intracranial pressure.

2 – f

Different anti-emetics are useful in different situations:

- Vomiting due to drugs – use haloperidol
- Vomiting due to gastric compression – use metoclopramide or domperidone
- Vomiting due to constipation – use an aperient
- Vomiting due to raised ICP – use steroids
- Vomiting due to bowel obstruction – drip and suck and either surgery as needed or octreotide and dexamethasone for small bowel obstruction

3 – e

Non-steroidal anti-inflammatory drugs are very useful for managing pain of bony origin. If the pain is from a metastasis, radiotherapy is an effective treatment.

System Module A: Locomotor System

Questions

1	Around the wrist	113
2	Lower limb nerve injuries	115
3	Management of open fractures	117
4	The shoulder	119
5	Bone diseases	121
6	Fractures of the femur	123
7	Child with a limp	125
8	The knee	127
9	Brachial Plexus injuries	129
10	Bone cysts and neoplasms	131

Question 1:
Theme: Around the wrist

Options:

    a   Colles' fracture
    b   Smith's fracture
    c   De Quervain's tenosynovitis
    d   Carpal tunnel syndrome
    e   Fractured scaphoid
    f   Bennett's fracture
    g   Barton's fracture
    h   Ganglion

For each of the patients described below, select the single most likely diagnosis from the options listed above. Each option may be used once, more than once or not at all.

1. A 70-year-old woman slips on ice while shopping and falls onto her outstretched left hand. She presents to casualty with an obviously deformed and tender wrist. X-rays reveal a completely fractured distal radius with volar angulation, carrying the carpus with it. The fracture line runs into the wrist joint.

2. A 40-year-old right-handed graphic designer presents to clinic complaining of a long history of worsening pain at the base of his right thumb. He does not recall any trauma. Examination reveals an area of maximal tenderness at the tip of the right radial styloid, which feels thicker than the left. Finkelstein's test is positive.

3. A 26-year-old woman presents with a painful and swollen hand having fallen while skiing. Her thumb was caught in the ice as she fell, and pain is maximal at its base on examination.

Question I: Answers

1 – g
Falling on to an outstretched hand usually causes different types of fracture depending upon the victim's age.

- Children – supracondylar fracture of the humerus
- Adults – fractured scaphoid
- Elderly – Colles' fracture

A **Colles'** fracture of the distal radius produces: 1, dorsal angulation; 2, radial deviation; and 3, impaction of the distal fragment. Treatment: reduction and below elbow plaster cast.

A **Smith's** fracture of the distal radius produces volar (anterior) angulation distally. Treatment: reduction and above elbow plaster cast.

A **Barton's** fracture has the distal radius fracture: 1, **extending into the joint line** with, 2, anterior angulation that angulates the attached **carpus anteriorly** also. Treatment: reduction and internal fixation with a small anterior plate is recommended as this **fracture–dislocation** is unstable.

A comminuted fracture involving the joint in the active patient may require an external fixator.

2 – c
De Quervain's tenosynovitis is inflammation of the sheath over the tendons forming the bottom of the anatomical snuffbox: extensor pollicis brevis (EPB) and abductor pollicis longus (APL). This is usually due to prolonged unusual or repetitive activity in the wrist (though the classic is in gardeners pruning roses). A positive Finkelstein's test is pain on forceful ulnar deviation of the wrist (thumb held in palm, or in a fist). There may also be pain on active extension against resistance (best done with the terminal phalanx of the thumb flexed).

A small cut under local anaesthesia will relieve pressure in the sheath, but surgeons must remember that the APL tendon is often a double tendon, and both parts will need to be cut to cure symptoms. Therefore, it is prudent to do Finkelstein's in theatre, after your initial tendon incision, to ensure you have relieved the patient's symptoms.

3 – f
Bennett's fracture is a fracture of the base of the thumb metacarpal that extends obliquely into the first carpometacarpal joint. If the large distal fragment displaces proximally, this produces a fracture–subluxation, which is difficult to stabilize. Treatment, therefore, is to pin the fracture with a small screw (and a plaster slab for 3 weeks).

Question 2:
Theme: Lower limb nerve injuries

Options:

- a Common peroneal nerve
- b Superficial peroneal nerve
- c Deep peroneal nerve
- d Tibial nerve
- e Sural nerve
- f Saphenous nerve
- g Sciatic nerve
- h Obturator nerve

For each of the cases described below, select the single most likely nerve at risk of injury from the options listed above. Each option may be used once, more than once or not at all.

1. A 34-year-old man visits a follow-up clinic with a high-stepping gait, having recovered from an open reduction and internal fixation of a comminuted fracture of his left tibia. On examination no muscle wasting is evident, ankle plantarflexion is normal, dorsiflexion is weak and ankle eversion is normal.

2. A 58-year-old woman undergoes an elective osteotomy to correct a hammer second toe of her right foot. She now complains of decreased sensation between her right big toe and second toe.

3. While crossing the road, a 15-year-old boy is hit on the lateral aspect of his left knee by a car. There is gross swelling around the head of his fibula, which is tender. Power is reduced in ipsilateral ankle dorsiflexion and ankle eversion.

Question 2: Answers

1 – c

2 – c

3 – a

Anatomically, the thigh extends from hip to knee, and the **leg** reaches from the knee to ankle. The **leg** is thus supplied **solely** by branches of the sciatic nerve (see diagram below and page 142).

(The femoral nerve supplies the anterior compartment of thigh and the obturator nerve supplies the adductor compartment. These nerves peter out at the knee and **do not** pass through the adductor hiatus into the popliteal fossa with the femoral artery and vein.)

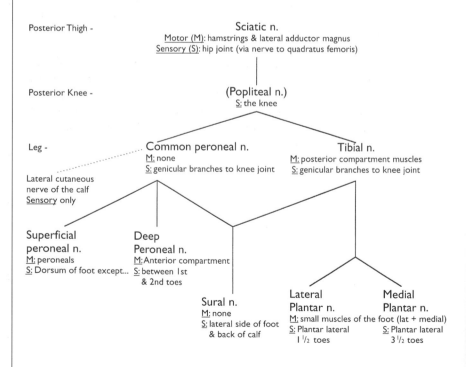

Posterior Thigh -

Sciatic n.
Motor (M): hamstrings & lateral adductor magnus
Sensory (S): hip joint (via nerve to quadratus femoris)

Posterior Knee -

(Popliteal n.)
S: the knee

Leg -

Common peroneal n.
M: none
S: genicular branches to knee joint

Tibial n.
M: posterior compartment muscles
S: genicular branches to knee joint

Lateral cutaneous
nerve of the calf
Sensory only

Superficial peroneal n.
M: peroneals
S: Dorsum of foot except...

Deep Peroneal n.
M: Anterior compartment
S: between 1st & 2nd toes

Sural n.
M: none
S: lateral side of foot & back of calf

Lateral Plantar n.
M: small muscles of the foot (lat + medial)
S: Plantar lateral 1 ½ toes

Medial Plantar n.
S: Plantar lateral 3 ½ toes

Question 3:
Theme: Management of open fractures

Options:

  a   Intravenous antibiotics only
  b   Debride, reduce, splint and leave open
  c   Debride, reduce, splint and close wound
  d   Debride, reduce, leave open and externally fixate
  e   Debride, reduce, leave open and internally fixate
  f   Reduction and back-slab plaster only
  g   Reduction and plaster cylinder only

For each of the patients described below, select the single most likely treat-ment from the options listed above. Each option may be used once, more than once or not at all.

1. A 24-year-old doctor fell off his motorbike 20 min ago while travel-ling at ~40 mph. He sustained an open, severely comminuted frac-ture of his tibia and fibula. He has no other significant injuries and has been adequately resuscitated. The wound on the leg is 12 cm long and contains some tarmac.

2. A 34-year-old farmer fell off his tractor landing on the plough behind. It has taken him 12 h to reach hospital. Examination reveals a 6 cm dirty wound and tender, swollen lower leg. X-rays demonstrate complete oblique fractures of his tibia and fibula with angulation. He has been adequately resuscitated in the Accident and Emergency Department.

Question 3: Answers

1 – d

2 – d

Management of open fractures is often open to debate, but certain principles can be applied.

- **R**esuscitate
- **A**nalgesia, **A**ntibiotics and **T**etanus
- **R**educe
- **R**ush to theatre
- **R**igorously wash out the wound (pulse irrigation) and debride devitalized tissue
- **R**eally low priority for use of a drain (from the most dependent part of the wound)

Three grades of open fracture exist:

- **Grade 1** – small, clean wound with minor soft-tissue damage
- **Grade 2** – wound > 1 cm with only moderate soft-tissue damage
- **Grade 3** – large wound with severe soft-tissue damage and contamination

- If the wound is small and is operated on in **< 6 h**, one may consider closure of skin and/or a skin graft
- All other wounds must be left open

Though grade 1 + 2 open fractures may be treated in much the same way as closed fractures, grade 3 fractures are most safely treated by external fixation (internal fixation is at greater risk of infection in these cases). **There is no rush anatomically to reduce a fracture. If the wound is grossly contaminated it is better to leave open, give intravenous antibiotics and fix the fracture in a few days.**

In general, **external fixation** is used:

- When there is severe soft-tissue injury
- Where the wound requires inspection
- Significant nerve or blood vessel damage has occurred
- For severely comminuted fractures
- Unstable fractures
- Pelvic fractures
- Infected fractures

Question 4:
Theme: The shoulder

Options:

- a   Chronic supraspinatus calcification (tendonitis)
- b   Supraspinatus partial tear
- c   Supraspinatus complete tear
- d   Septic arthritis
- e   Osteomyelitis
- f   Frozen shoulder
- g   Long thoracic nerve palsy
- h   Anterior dislocation of shoulder
- i   Posterior dislocation of shoulder

For each of the clinical vignettes described below, select the single most likely diagnosis from the options listed above. Each option may be used once, more than once or not at all.

1. A 46-year-old man presents with an acutely tender right shoulder. He does not recall any trauma. On examination the arm is held in medial rotation with markedly decreased movement due to pain. He is also bleeding from a bitten tongue. An A-P radiograph appears normal, but the lateral view is conclusive.

2. A 52-year-old window cleaner presents to his general practitioner complaining of an aching shoulder. The pain is always worst at night. Recently, the pain has been very severe when trying to put on a shirt or jacket. On examination the acromion is tender, and abduction is painful with the forearm in the neutral position, but not with the arm in full external rotation.

3. A 40-year-old ex-professional javelin thrower presents to the Accident and Emergency Department with acute right shoulder pain. It occurred while lifting some weights at a gym this morning, but now he can not lift his arm above his head. The A&E registrar has injected some local anaesthetic into the joint, and when you come to see the patient he can move his shoulder fully with no pain. There is some crepitus felt over the shoulder joint with abduction.

Question 4: Answers

1 – i

The rotator cuff is deficient inferiorly. Dislocations of the humeral head from the glenoid cavity will cause the acromion to be the most lateral point, as opposed to the humeral head, which causes the 'squared off' appearance of the shoulder. Posterior dislocations are far less common and produce a characteristic 'light-bulb sign' on an A-P X-ray film and, if not paying attention, can look normal on A-P radiographs. Thus, the lateral view is all-important in distinguishing an anterior from a posterior dislocation. Though rare, one must always consider a posterior dislocation of the shoulder after an epileptic fit (as in this case) or an electric shock.

2 – a

The rotator cuff muscles comprise **'SITS': supraspinatus, infraspinatus, teres minor and subscapularis.**

Arising from the scapula, the first three insert as a conjoint tendon into the greater tuberosity of the humerus and subscapularis into the lesser tuberosity. They act to keep the head of the humerus firmly in the glenoid whenever the arm is lifted by deltoid. The fibro-osseous **coraco-acromial arch** keeps them from springing upwards (separated by the subacromial bursa).

With age, the cuff degenerates and repair causes calcification, especially at the relatively avascular supraspinatus insertion. It is probably the sub-acute or chronic vascular reaction to calcification that causes supraspinatus tendonitis. This produces a '**painful arc**' between 60 and 120°, as the inflamed area is caught against the coraco-acromial ligament. External rotation moves supraspinatus posterior to the arch, and stops it getting trapped. This is a virtually pathagnomonic sign.

3 – b

In the acute phase, both partial and complete rotator cuff tears impede abduction. They can be distinguished because a patient with a **partial** tear will be able to abduct after a local anaesthetic injection has been given in to the painful area. A partial tear requires rest and analgesia, whereas a complete tear can not be fixed without surgery. Crepitus or clicking suggests a partial tear of the rotator cuff.

A **complete** tear will present acutely, and the patient will be unable to abduct his arm actively and can only manage a characteristic shoulder shrug. However, if abducted > 90° **passively**, it will stay in place due to the action of deltoid (the 'abduction paradox'). When lowered, it falls suddenly (the 'drop arm sign').

Question 5:
Theme: Bone diseases

Options:

  a Osteoporosis
  b Osteomalacia
  c Paget's disease
  d Primary hyperparathyroidism
  e Multiple myeloma

For each of the set of results described below, select the single most likely diagnosis from the options listed above. Each option may be used once, more than once or not at all.

	Ca^{2+} (total) mmol/L^{-1}	PO_4 mmol/L^{-1}	ALP IUl^{-1}
1	2.4	1.1	200
2	2.3	1.4	640

Normal values:

- Ca^{2+} (total) = 2.12–2.65 mmol/L^{-1}
- PO_4 = 0.8–1.45 mmol/L^{-1}
- ALP = 30–300 IU/L^{-1}

Question 5: Answers

1 – a

2 – c

The main biochemical differences between bone diseases are sum-
marised as:

Disease	Ca^{2+}	PO_4	ALP	PTH
Osteomalacia/rickets*	Tends to be ↓	↔, ↓	↔, ↑	↑
Paget's disease	↔	↔	↑↑↑	↔
Osteoporosis	↔	↔	↔	↔
Osteosclerosis	↔	↔	↔	↑
Renal osteodystrophy	↓	↑	↔	↑↑
Bone metastases	↑, ↓, ↔	↑, ↓, ↔	↑, ↔	↓
Primary hyperparathyroidism	↑	↓, ↔	↑	↑

*25-Hydroxycholecalciferol will be decreased if the disease is due to vitamin D defi-
ciency

Question 6:
Theme: Fractures of the femur

Options:

    a   Hemi-arthroplasty
    b   Total hip replacement
    c   Arthrodesis
    d   Dynamic hip screw
    e   Cannulated screws
    f   Full leg plaster cylinder

For each of the fractures described below, select the single most likely treatment from the options listed above. Each option may be used once, more than once or not at all.

1. A 78-year-old woman falls out of bed. An X-ray reveals an undisplaced intertrochanteric fractured neck of femur.

2. A 45-year-old man is hit on the thigh by a van. X-ray investigation shows an intracapsular fractured neck of femur that is minimally displaced.

3. A 77-year-old woman trips on a loose patio stone in her garden and is now complaining of left hip pain. She could previously mobilise for a maximum of ~20 metres with a stick, but is unable to weight bear now. X-ray investigation reveals a Garden IV intracapsular fracture.

Question 6: Answers

1 – d

The main principle behind fractured neck of femur fractures is to conserve blood supply to the neck of the femur.

An **intra**capsular (as opposed to **extra**-) fracture puts the femoral head at risk of avascular necrosis in the elderly, as it will disrupt the retinacular vessels and nutrient artery supply, leaving only the inadequate artery in the ligamentum teres. The Garden classification:

- **Garden I – Uni**cortical fracture with femoral head undisplaced on neck
- **Garden II – Bi**cortical fracture; neck **un**displaced
- **Garden III –** Head **partially** displaced; trabeculae **un**aligned across fracture site
- **Garden IV –** Head **completely** displaced; trabeculae disrupted

Then use the following rhyme to determine treatment:

- Garden I and II – **cannulated screw**
- Garden III and IV – **Austin–Moore**

Intertrochanteric fractures (which are extracapsular) unite easily and seldom cause avascular necrosis. A **dynamic hip screw** allows gradual collapse of the femoral head. They are not used for intracapsular fractures as the head would spin around the axis of the screw and ruin its blood supply.

2 – e

Younger patients will have a better blood supply to the head of femur and therefore one can consider cannulated screws for internal fixation of even intracapsular fractures as the joint will be **preserved**. By having three screws, the femoral head is prevented from spinning around its axis, compromising blood supply (the same principle applies for a DHS + derotational screw).

3 – a

In elderly patients it is desirable to perform the quickest and easiest operation to return them to their previous state of health. If left untreated, almost 30% of these patients die within 3 months from the lack of mobility causing pneumonia, DVT, bedsores and UTIs.

Hemi-arthroplasty (e.g. with an Austin–Moore prosthesis) is a quick and less complicated operation than total hip replacement (THR). It is performed in the elderly (e.g. > 70 years) as they tend to have co-morbid illnesses making their tolerance for major surgery poor. It is used in those who have poor mobility normally, as they are less likely to wear away the acetabular cartilage surface with their new metal prosthesis.

If the patient is younger (e.g. 60–70 years), fit for major surgery or cannulated screws have already failed, one may consider THR. Similarly, a fit elderly patient with a grossly degenerate acetabular surface may be considered for THR.

Avascular necrosis can occur up to 2 years after surgery. Therefore, follow-up ought to be for this length of time with at-risk patients, i.e. those that have cannulated screws inserted.

Question 7:
Theme: Child with a limp

Options:
- a   Perthe's disease
- b   Slipped upper femoral epiphysis (SUFE)
- c   Septic arthritis
- d   Rheumatoid arthritis
- e   Congenital dislocation of the hip (CDH)
- f   Transient synovitis

For each of the clinical vignettes described below, select the single most likely diagnosis from the options listed above. Each option may be used once, more than once or not at all.

1. A mother brings her 2-year-old daughter to her general practitioner stating that her daughter seems to limp due to a short left leg. On examination, the leg is not tender, the groin skin creases are asymmetrical and the hip does not abduct fully. Measuring the true leg length reveals a shortened left leg, which is slightly externally rotated. The Trendelenburg test is positive.

2. A 6-year-old boy presents to clinic having been referred by his general practitioner for an acutely painful right hip. There is no history of trauma or birth difficulties. He is of medium height, slightly plump and the hip looks normal. Hip movements are now full, with the exception of abduction and internal rotation, whereas when he presented to his general practitioner all hip movements were limited and painful at the extremes of movement. Radioisotope scanning reveals a void in the right head of femur.

3. A 12-year-old girl complains of a 1-week history of right hip pain. There is no history of trauma and X-rays reveal no abnormality. Examination is unremarkable. One week later, with bed rest and NSAID, the pain has completely resolved with no restriction of leg movement.

Question 7: Answers

1 – e

This is a late presentation of CDH – now known as developmental dysplasia of the hip (DDH). Screening at birth with Ortolani's or Barlow's test should successfully screen for this disorder, which usually resolves spontaneously within 3 weeks, but persistently affects 2/1000 births. It has a higher incidence in breech deliveries and intrauterine malposition.

In late cases, X-rays reveal an upward sloping acetabular roof with a shallow socket. The femoral head is displaced upwards and outwards and the ossification centre of the femoral head is underdeveloped.

2 – a

The case describes Perthe's disease. A 'void' on radioisotope scanning appears before X-ray changes. The earliest X-ray changes are increased density of the bone epiphysis and apparent widening of the joint space. Later, the femoral head appears flattened, with lateral displacement of the epiphysis and then rarefaction and broadening of the metaphysis.

SUFE causes an A-P X-ray to have a wide epiphysis and a line drawn along the superior surface of the femoral neck continues superior to the head rather than passing through it (Trethowan's sign).

3 – f

This is a classic story of transient synovitis, which is a differential diagnosis of Perthe's disease. Ultrasound may show a joint effusion and treatment is bed rest and analgesia until the effusion resolves.

In general, the aetiology of hip pain can usually be diagnosed by the age at which it presents (with a few exceptions, e.g. juvenile arthritis).

Age (years)	Probable diagnosis
0 (birth)	CDH
0–5	Infection
5–10	Perthe's disease
10–20	SUFE
Adults	Osteoarthitis; avascular necrosis; rheumatoid arthritis

The reason for Perthe's occurring between 5 and 10 years is because this is the age at which the retinacular and nutrient arteries take over from the artery in ligamentum teres from being the main blood supply to the femoral head. A mismatch causes the avascular changes of Perthe's.

SUFE occurs during the adolescent growth spurt, typically in children who are very tall or very fat with abnormal gonadal development. It is thus thought possibly due to an imbalance of pituitary growth hormone (for bone growth) and gonadal hormone (for physeal fusion), which result in a weak physis. This will explain trauma causing an 'acute on chronic' slip.

Question 8:
Theme: The knee

Options:
    a   Medial meniscal tear
    b   Anterior cruciate ligament tear
    c   Posterior cruciate ligament tear
    d   Patellar tendon rupture
    e   Lateral collateral ligament tear
    f   Medial collateral ligament tear

For each of the cases described below, select the single most likely diagnosis from the options listed above. Each option may be used once, more than once or not at all.

1. A 30-year-old man plays football and falls awkwardly in a tackle, resulting in a painful knee that becomes swollen over the next few hours. He rests it at home with some ice and recovers enough to play football again a fortnight later. However, during the match, he misses a kick and the same knee twists as the foot is planted firmly in the ground. On examination, the knee is swollen with movement that is limited at the extreme of extension.

2. A 45-year-old woman driver is involved in a head-on collision between her car and a tree. Wearing her seatbelt, she sustains no obvious external injury but complains of a painful knee where it hit the dashboard. On examination, there is an effusion of her knee joint and the tibia appears to ride back on the femur.

Question 8: Answers

1 – a

This man has damaged his medial meniscus. The menisci are 'C'-shaped wedges of fibrocartilage that lie between the tibia and femur, one under each femoral condyle. They are most commonly damaged during twisting injuries of the knee.

It is far commoner to injure the medial than the lateral meniscus. This is because the medial meniscus is actually attached to the medial collateral ligament, which is stretched taut when the knee is twisted and may be damaged itself. The lateral meniscus is not attached to the lateral collateral ligament; in fact it is separated from it by the tendon of popliteus. It is therefore more mobile and less likely to be damaged.

It is important to differentiate between an injury to a meniscus and a cruciate ligament in the knee. If a ligament is torn, it will result in immediate swelling in the knee (haemarthrosis). Tearing of a comparatively avascular meniscus will swell the knee over a few hours. A torn meniscus may wedge in the knee joint and prevent it from fully extending, a phenomenon known as locking.

2 – c

The tibia of this unfortunate woman was violently posteriorly displaced on her femur, stretching and finally rupturing her posterior cruciate ligament. With her knees partially flexed, she will demonstrate the 'sag sign', in which the tibia will appear to sag lower down on the femur when compared with the other side.

Classic scenarios:

- Anterior cruciate ligament tear – knee gives going **upstairs**
- Posterior cruciate ligament tear – knee gives going **downstairs**

Question 9:
Theme: Brachial plexus injuries

Options:

    a   Upper trunk
    b   Lower trunk
    c   Fifth and sixth cervical roots
    d   Eighth cervical and first thoracic root
    e   Lateral cord
    f   Medial cord

For each of the cases described below, select the single most likely part of the brachial plexus that has been injured from the options listed above. Each option may be used once, more than once or not at all.

1. A 22-year-old motorcyclist is thrown off his bike in a road traffic accident and lands on his right side. On examination, his right arm is hanging limply by his side in medial rotation. Sensation is decreased on the outer arm forearm on that side and there is no winging of his scapulae.

2. During an argument with his wife in the kitchen, a 37-year-old man is stabbed at the base of the posterior triangle of his neck on the left side. He subsequently develops a hand with fixed hyperextension at the metacarpophalangeal joints and flexion at the interphalangeal joints with a Horner's syndrome on that side. He has diminished sensation on the medial side of his forearm and on the little finger ipsilaterally.

Question 9: Answers

1 – a

Lesions to the upper brachial plexus usually occur when the head and shoulder on one side are forcibly pushed away from each other. Commonly this may happen to the newborn during childbirth, or after a rider falls off his motorbike. The subsequent lesion is described in the question and its appearance is that of a 'porter's tip'. The whole pattern of injury is called an 'Erb–Duchenne palsy'.

The upper brachial plexus is formed by the C5 and C6 roots. The lower brachial plexus is formed by the C8 and T1 roots. A C5–6 **root** injury will cause paralysis of the scapular muscles and anaesthesia over the area of the back supplied by the C5 and C6 dorsal primary rami. The long thoracic nerve will also be affected, causing paralysis of serratus anterior and therefore winging of the scapula.

An upper trunk injury will spare the long thoracic nerve.

2 – d

The knife has divided the C8 and T1 nerve roots. The T1 root is of special interest as it supplies all of the small muscles of the hand. It is also the first place from which sympathetic nerve fibres leave the spinal cord. These preganglionic fibres will travel in the T1 nerve root and leave almost immediately to synapse with the post-ganglionic fibres, some of which will then travel upwards to supply the whole of the head and neck.

Damage to the preganglionic part of the T1 root will prevent sympathetic outflow from reaching the eye on that side, and therefore will cause a unilateral Horner's syndrome.

The Brachial Plexus (main branches only):

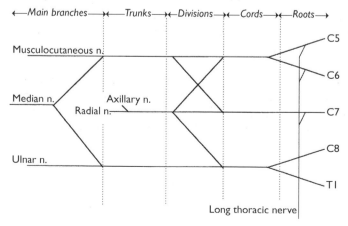

Question 10:
Theme: Bone cysts and neoplasms

Options:

a   Osteoid osteoma
b   Chondroma
c   Giant cell tumour
d   Bone cyst
e   Osteoclastoma
f   Ewing's sarcoma
g   Fibrosarcoma
h   Chondrosarcoma
i   Multiple myeloma
j   Osteosarcoma

For each of the patients described below, select the single most likely diagnosis from the options listed above. Each option may be used once, more than once or not at all.

1. A 13-year-old boy complains of pain in his left knee, which has been gradually increasing in severity over a few weeks. It is constant and keeps him awake at night. The overlying skin is warm and shiny. X-ray of the knee reveals bone destruction in the metaphysis of his left femur, with areas of new bone formation and periosteal elevation.

2. A 16-year-old boy complains of a painful shoulder after a particularly physical tackle during a rugby match. Examination reveals focal tenderness just below the head of the humerus and movement limited by pain. X-rays reveal a spherical radiolucent area with a clearly demarcated smooth edge in the metaphysis that extends into, but not beyond, the cortical margins which have retained their normal outer contour. There is a new fracture running through it. He has never had any shoulder pain previously.

3. A 15-year-old boy complains of an ache in his upper arm. There is no history of trauma. On examination he is apyrexial and has a hot, hard swelling in the middle of his arm. X-rays demonstrate an onion skin-shaped bone lesion in the medulla of his humerus.

Question 10: Answers

1 – j
This patient has an osteosarcoma of his left femur. These highly malignant lesions appear in two age groups: between 10 and 20 years, and also in the > 50s secondary to Paget's disease.

Osteosarcomas usually occur at the metaphysis of long bones and present with pain, often after a history of trauma. The periosteal new bone formation produces a speckled triangle (Codman's triangle) on the X-ray; this is known as 'sun-ray spiculation'.

Resectable tumours are treated with cytotoxic therapy, followed by surgical resection. There is now a 50% 5-year survival rate.

2 – d
Bone cysts are painless and can cause a pathological fracture at any time in life. However, they usually present up to the age of puberty. They appear as a radiolucent (black) sphere on X-ray, usually on the side of a long bone metaphysis. (Differential diagnosis: fibrous cortical defect).

Osteoid osteomas are painful and have a sclerotic rim. As cysts are rare in adults, it is thought that most spontaneously regress. Injection of corticosteroids into a cyst may obliterate them, though one may also curette the inside and fill with bone chips. Note that aneurysmal bone cysts are more likely to expand the cortex (and therefore look like giant cell tumours) and they are confined to the metaphyseal side of the growth plate.

3 – f
Ewing's sarcoma is a rare malignant tumour of bone. It presents in long bone medullary cavities, between 10 and 30 years of age and is believed to derive from vascular endothelium in bone marrow. Osteomyelitis is a differential diagnosis. Despite treatment with radiotherapy, chemotherapy or even amputation, the survival rate at 5 years is 35%.

System Module B: Vascular

Questions

1	Lower limb vascular disease	135
2	Lower limb amputation	137
3	Treatment of arterial occlusion	139
4	Anatomy of the lower limb	141
5	Aneurysms	143
6	Upper limb anatomy	145
7	Splenomegaly	147
8	Leg ulcers	149
9	Aortic aneurysms	151
10	Carotid endarterectomy	153

Question 1:
Theme: Lower limb vascular disease

Options:

    a Acute ischaemia of the foot
    b Popliteal artery occlusion
    c Profunda femoris occlusion
    d Leriche's syndrome
    e Phlegmasia alba dolens
    f Phlegmasia cerulea dolens

For each of the patients described below, select the single most likely diagnosis from the options listed above. Each option may be used once, more than once or not at all.

1. A 63-year-old male smoker complains of a gradually worsening history of pain in the buttocks on walking. He has recently become impotent. On examination he has pale cold legs. The femoral pulses are absent on both sides.

2. A 59-year-old woman complains of cramping in her right calf when she walks uphill. It is relieved by standing still for 1 min.

3. A 26-year-old woman who is 34/40 weeks pregnant develops a painful and hot right leg with dilatation of the superficial veins. The leg becomes oedematous and turns milky white in colour.

Question I: Answers

1 – d

This patient has occlusion of the terminal aorta. This results in a reduced flow to the external iliac artery (which becomes the femoral artery and supplies the leg), as well as to the internal iliac artery (which will supply the pelvis and perineum).

The result is a bilateral buttock claudication with impotence, otherwise known as Leriche's syndrome.

2 – b

The popliteal artery is a direct continuation of the femoral artery as it passes from the front of the thigh through adductor magnus and into the popliteal fossa behind. Occlusion here will restrict blood to the limb below the knee joint and cause intermittent claudication of the calf.

3 – e

Pelvic masses, including a gravid uterus, may cause a deep venous thrombosis (DVT). If a DVT is high or large enough it will obstruct the return of blood from the **deep** venous system of the leg. The leg will then become hot and the superficial veins will dilate, but the eventual oedema will turn the leg milky white. This is known as phlegmasia alba dolens, and classically occurs with massive pelvic vein thrombosis. The leg is warm as the arterial supply is still present.

If **all** of the main veins become obstructed due to a DVT, the skin becomes congested and turns blue. This appearance is called phlegmasia cerulea dolens, and it signifies impending venous gangrene.

Question 2:
Theme: Lower limb amputation

Options:

  a   Above knee amputation
  b   Through knee amputation
  c   Below knee amputation
  d   Symes amputation
  e   Transmetatarsal amputation

For each of the descriptions below, select the single most likely amputation from the options listed above. Each option may be used once, more than once or not at all.

1. This amputation is used to remove diabetic gangrene of the toes.

2. This amputation goes as low as possible through the distal tibia and fibula.

3. The amputation is covered with equal sized anterior and posterior skin flaps.

Question 2: Answers

1 – e
The small vessel disease of diabetes results in toe ischaemia with relatively good blood supply to the surrounding tissues. Necrotic toes may be individually removed with a ray amputation, or may be collectively removed via a transmetatarsal amputation.

2 – d
In a Syme's amputation, the surgeon will try to preserve as much of the tibia and fibula as possible with removal of the mortice joint of the ankle.

3 – a
The skin below the knee joint has a poor blood supply anteriorly and is liable to break down after the operation. Therefore, a long posterior or skew flap (which are well vascularised) are used to overcome this problem. As this problem is less likely above the knee, equal-sized anterior and posterior skin flaps may be used.

Through-knee amputations are usually used in children where one is aiming to maintain the growth plate; it is rarely used for ischaemic surgery.

Question 3:
Theme: Treatment of arterial occlusion

Options:

    a   Thrombolysis
    b   Femoro-popliteal bypass
    c   Heparinization only
    d   Amputation
    e   Conservative treatment
    f   Angioplasty
    g   Embolectomy

For each of the clinical scenarios described below, select the single most likely management from the options listed above. Each option may be used once, more than once or not at all.

1. A 64-year-old man presents with a painful cold foot. He has an absent right popliteal pulse and no pedal pulses. Urgent arteriography demonstrates a thrombosed popliteal aneurysm with no run off.

2. A 67-year-old woman is known to have calf claudication. She stopped smoking 4 years ago, but despite this her symptoms gradually deteriorated. She now regularly wakes at night with pain in her right calf, which is relieved by hanging her leg over the edge of her bed. Her arteriogram shows a long occlusion in her superficial femoral artery.

3. A 41-year-old tourist from Australia develops sudden left-sided pleuritic chest pain 2 days into her holiday in London. Her oxygen saturation is 96% on air, and a V/Q scan demonstrates a small mismatch in the left lower lobe.

Question 3: Answers

1 – a
A thrombosed popliteal aneurysm is an indication for thrombolysis. The acutely ischaemic leg may be due to either thrombosis of an existing atheroma, or an embolus. See diagram for treatment options.

2 – b
The natural history of intermittent claudication is that:

- One-third gets better within 1–2 years
- One-third stays the same
- One-third gets worse

The typical pattern of progression is from:

- **Claudication → rest pain → gangrene**

A patient who presents with intermittent claudication should give up smoking first (they inevitably do smoke!). Associated diseases should be controlled, and a gradual exercise programme instigated. This develops the collateral circulation.

The ankle/brachial pressure index (ABPI) must be measured. Angiography is performed either at presentation or if the condition worsens. If this demonstrates a short occlusion, one can proceed to angioplasty (balloon, sub-intimal or stent) during the investigation. A long occlusion, or failure of angioplasty needs bypass surgery.

- Claudication occurs at ABPI **< 0.7**
- Rest pain occurs at ABPI **< 0.4**
- Critical ischaemia occurs at ABPI **< 0.3**

3 – c
Thrombolysis is only indicated in **large** pulmonary emboli, i.e. one that causes hypoxia. Note that this flow diagram is a guide only:

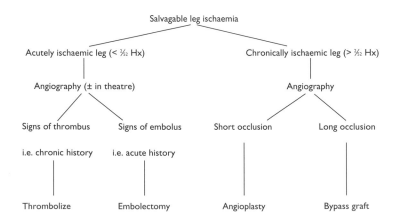

Question 4:
Theme: Anatomy of the lower limb

Options:

- a   Pectineus
- b   Piriformis
- c   Adductor magnus
- d   Adductor longus
- e   Adductor brevis
- f   Biceps femoris
- g   Sural nerve
- h   Saphenous nerve
- i   Lateral plantar nerve

For each of the descriptions below, select the single most likely anatomical structure from the options listed above. Each option may be used once, more than once or not at all.

1. This forms a boundary of the femoral triangle.

2. The sciatic nerve lies on this in the thigh.

3. Damage during short saphenous varicose vein surgery causes tingling in the little toe.

Question 4: Answers

1 – d
The femoral triangle:

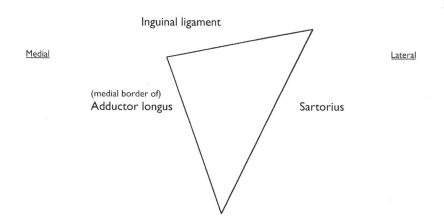

Inguinal ligament

Medial

Lateral

(medial border of)
Adductor longus

Sartorius

- **Floor** (lateral to medial) – iliacus, psoas, pectineus, adductor longus
- **Roof** – skin and fascial layers
- **Contents** (lateral to medial) – femoral nerve, femoral artery, femoral vein, femoral canal (containing the lymphatics).

2 – c
The **sciatic** nerve appears from under piriformis. Its surface marking is half way between the ischial tuberosity and greater trochanter. It then travels down the thigh on adductor magnus and is crossed by the long head of biceps femoris.

3 – g
The **sural** nerve accompanies the short saphenous nerve on the calf and both dive behind the lateral malleolus. It is sensory to the lateral side of the dorsum of the foot (as well as the back of the calf).

The **saphenous** nerve accompanies the great saphenous vein anterior to the medial malleolus and is sensory to the dorsum of the medial aspect of the foot (as well as the medial side of the calf). **All other motor and sensory nerves below the knee arise from the sciatic nerve.**

See page 116.

Question 5:
Theme: Aneurysms

Options:

    a   Mycotic aneurysm
    b   Congenital aneurysm
    c   False aneurysm
    d   Dissecting aneurysm
    e   Degenerative aneurysm

For each of the patients described below, select the single most likely type of aneurysm from the options listed above. Each option may be used once, more than once or not at all.

1. A previously well 26-year-old man complains of a sudden 'thunder-clap' headache. He dies on the way to hospital.

2. A 66-year-old man undergoes an aortic valve replacement. One year later he develops fevers and pain behind the right knee. A pulsatile mass can be felt in the right popliteal fossa.

3. A pulsating groin lump is felt in a patient the day after arterial blood gas sampling is performed from the femoral artery on that side.

Question 5: Answers

1 – b
This patient died of a ruptured Berry aneurysm, which is a congenital abnormality. Other congenital aneurysms may be due to Marfan's or Ehlers–Danlos syndrome.

2 – a
A mycotic aneurysm is due to infection. In our patient this was secondary to bacterial endocarditis. The classic example is of thoracic aortic aneurysm secondary to syphilis.

3 – c
A false aneurysm follows trauma. It is 'false' because the wall of the aneurysm is actually the edge of a haematoma, which is in direct connection with the lumen of the blood vessel from which it arose. It is more common in anticoagulated patients, or those with clotting disorders.

Question 6:
Theme: Upper limb anatomy

Options:

- a   Axillary nerve
- b   Radial artery
- c   Axillary artery
- d   Median nerve
- e   Tendon of biceps brachii
- f   Radial nerve
- g   Brachial artery

For each of the descriptions below, select the single most likely anatomical structure from the options listed above. Each option may be used once, more than once or not at all.

1. This structure passes through the quadrilateral space.

2. This structure is found lateral to the brachial artery in the cubital fossa.

3. This structure runs in the spiral groove.

4. This structure can be easily palpated in the anatomical snuffbox.

Question 6: Answers

1 – a
The quadrilateral space is formed by the humerus laterally, the long head of triceps medially, teres minor above and teres major below. The axillary nerve and posterior circumflex artery of the humerus pass through it.

2 – e
In the cubital fossa, the brachial artery is surrounded by the median nerve medially and the tendon of biceps brachii laterally.

3 – f
The radial nerve runs in the spiral groove on the posterior aspect of the humerus between the medial and lateral heads of triceps. It may be damaged by a mid-shaft fracture of the humerus, or by falling asleep with one's arm draped over the back of a chair – the so called 'Saturday night palsy'. The patient will suffer a wrist drop, with triceps function preserved. Sensory loss is classically over the first dorsal interosseous muscle, but may extend to a small strip of skin on the posterior aspect of the forearm and arm.

4 – b
Anatomical snuffbox:

- Boundaries:
    - Posteriorly – Extensor pollicis longus
    - Anteriorly – Extensor pollicis brevis
                             Abductor pollicis longus

- Floor (proximal to distal):
    - Styloid process of the radius
    - Scaphoid bone
    - Trapezium and base of the first metacarpal bone

- Contents:
    - Radial artery (runs ventral to dorsal)
    - Tendons of extensor carpi radialis longus and brevis
    - Radial nerve (cutaneous branches)
    - Cephalic vein

- Roof:
    - Skin
    - Fascial layers

Question 7:
Theme: Splenomegaly

Options:

   a   Infectious mononucleosis
   b   Portal hypertension
   c   Chronic granulocytic leukaemia
   d   Malaria
   e   Brucellosis
   f   Felty's syndrome
   g   Amyloid
   h   Spherocytosis
   i   Polycythaemia vera
   j   Sickle cell anaemia

For each of the cases described below, select the single most likely diagnosis from the options listed above. Each option may be used once, more than once or not at all.

1. A 27-year-old Irish man presents with malaise, enlarged tonsils and splenomegaly. He has a positive monospot test result.

2. A 15-year-old Scottish girl has a 9-month history of generalised joint aches, with decreased mobility. On examination, she has a bilateral symmetrical destructive polyarthropathy and splenomegaly.

3. A 16-year-old Welsh girl presents with right upper quadrant pain. She appears mildly jaundiced and has mild splenomegaly. Ultrasound of her abdomen reveals gallstones.

Question 7: Answers

1 – a

2 – f
Felty's syndrome is chronic rheumatoid arthritis with splenomegaly.

3 – h
Hereditary spherocytosis occurs as a genetic defect alters the red cell membrane. The abnormally shaped corpuscles become trapped in the splenic microcirculation and die. This causes splenomegaly, and the resulting breakdown of haemoglobin causes anaemia and jaundice. Bile pigment is derived from the breakdown of haemoglobin, and gallstones are therefore more likely to form.

Causes of splenomegaly:

Massive (past the umbilicus)	Moderate (up to the umbilicus)	Mild (just palpable)
Chronic granulocytic leukaemia	Chronic lymphocytic leukaemia	Felty's syndrome (rheumatoid arthritis)
Myelofibrosis	Portal hypertension	Amyloid
Kala–Azar	Lymphoma	Hepatitis
Sickle cell anaemia (in children before autosplenectomy)	Malaria	Infectious mononucleosis (Epstein–Barr virus)
	All the above may also cause mild splenomegaly	Polycythaemia rubra vera
		Spherocytosis
		SLE

Question 8:
Theme: Leg ulcers

Options:

a   Venous ulcer
b   Ischaemic ulcer
c   Malignant melanoma
d   Marjolin's ulcer
e   Basal cell carcinoma
f   Rheumatoid ulcer
g   Pyoderma gangrenosum
h   Systemic lupus erythematosus
i   Traumatic ulcer
j   Neuropathic ulcer (trophic ulcer)

For each of the cases described below, select the single most likely type of leg ulcer from the options listed above. Each option may be used once, more than once or not at all.

1. A 54-year-old woman presents with an ulcer over the anteromedial aspect of the lower limb. It is flat, with edges sloping towards the centre and has a seropurulent discharge. She does not recall any trauma. She has suffered 'for years' with an aching pain over the leg due to her varicose veins and has noted that this area seemed to have a brown discoloration over the past few months.

2. A 66-year-old man with insulin–dependent diabetes mellitus is noted to have an ulcer on the base of his left heel while being preclerked for laser surgery for his retinopathy.

3. A 50-year-old Caucasian woman notes a long standing 'raw spot' on her left lateral calf has slowly enlarged to 2 cm diameter over the past 2 months, and its edges seem to have become heaped up and turned dark red. It is now becoming tender and is oozing blood from its centre.

Question 8: Answers

1 – a
Venous ulcers are commonly secondary to venous stasis from varicose veins and/or DVT. They invariably begin after the skin of the leg has been knocked and damaged. However, the patient may not remember the initial insult.

2 – j
Neuropathic ulcers are caused by trauma (usually prolonged pressure) that is not perceived due to sensory loss; hence they occur over pressure-bearing areas.

3 – d
A chronic venous ulcer may rarely undergo metaplasia to form a squamous cell carcinoma, which is called a Marjolin's ulcer. Be suspicious if inguinal lymph nodes are palpable. A basal cell carcinoma has a raised white pearly edge.

Refer to the table to distinguish the commonest three types of ulcer:

	Arterial	Venous	Neuropathic
Site	Tips of toes and pressure areas	Lower third medial calf (usually): 'gaiter area'	Pressure sites: heels, fifth MT, ball of foot
Size	1 mm to 10 cm	Any	Any
Edge	Punched out (adjacent tissue cannot heal)	Sloping towards centre. Edges purple/blue	Punched out
Base	Sloughy or pale and flat (no blood supply for granulation)	Pink granulation with white fibrous tissue ± slough; **rarely** infected	Same as arterial
Pain	Yes	Declines with time	No (**characteristic**)
Depth	Deep (even to bone)	Shallow and flat	Deep
Discharge	Clear serum or pus; blood unlikely	Seropurulent with occasional blood	Same as arterial
Surrounding tissue	Cold, pallor, atrophy. Pulses absent	Warm	Anaesthesia. Pulses present Test PNS and CNS
General condition	?Sensory loss; test BM	Old women. Long Hx	
Causes	Arteriopathy*	Abnormal venous blood flow, e.g. after DVT or varicose veins	**Diabetes**, nerve lesions, leprosy, tabes dorsalis, spina bifida, syrinx
Treatment	Correct arteriopathy	Compression dressings Elevation	Protection from pressure

*Ischaemic ulceration:
- Large artery disease:
  - Atherosclerosis
  - Embolism
- Small artery disease:
  - **Pathology**:
    - Scleroderma
    - Buerger's disease
    - Embolism
    - Diabetes
    - Raynaud's disease
- **or Physical agents**:
  - Pressure necrosis
    - Radiation
    - Trauma
    - Electric burns

Question 9:
Theme: Aortic aneurysms

Options:
  a   Immediate endovascular stenting
  b   Immediate CT scan
  c   Check pulse and blood pressure hourly
  d   Insert two wide bore intravenous lines, crossmatch blood and transfer to theatre
  e   Immediate ultrasound
  f   Thrombolyse

For each of the patients described below, select the single most appropriate management from the options listed above. Each option may be used once, more than once or not at all.

1. A 68-year-old man presents with sudden back pain. He is pale with a heart rate = 120 beats min^{-1} and blood pressure = 80/40 mmHg. An epigastric mass is palpable and tender.

2. A 58-year-old man is admitted with thoracic back pain. He is noted to have a palpable expansile epigastric mass. His heart rate = 80 beats min^{-1} and blood pressure = 130/67 mmHg. Chest X-ray shows gross widening of his mediastinum.

Question 9: Answers

1 – d
Abdominal aortic aneurysms (AAA) with back pain and shock are **leak-ing.** They need immediate reconstructive surgery, as 50% of patients die before reaching hospital, and of those who arrive, 50% die either of shock before theatre or of acute renal failure after. Fluid resuscitate **carefully** (to avoid clot disruption and catastrophic leak from the aneurysm) and get to theatre!

A patient with any symptoms is at risk of imminent rupture and therefore needs surgery.

An **elective** operation has < 6% mortality rate. Thus, asymptomatic aneurysms (e.g. found on routine examination or noticed by the patient) are regularly followed up with ultrasound or CT scan. This is because an AAA with a diameter of > 6 cm has a 75% chance of rupture within 1 year. Therefore, most surgeons operate by the time the aneurysm reaches 5.5 cm in diameter.

2 – b
A patient with a widened mediastinum on chest X-ray needs to have a thoracic aortic aneurysm excluded. The gold standard investigation to detect this is angiography, but CT scanning is easier and non-invasive. Both will show whether the aneurysm is due to aortic dissection. This was a patient with the signs and symptoms of an aortic aneurysm, but he was stable and could therefore afford the time to have a CT scan rather than be rushed to theatre. A patient with one aneurysm has a > 25% chance of having one somewhere else – hence the epigastric mass in this case.

Question 10:
Theme: Carotid endarterectomy

Options:

a   Facial vein
b   Superior thyroid vein
c   Internal jugular vein
d   Omohyoid
e   Anterior belly of digastric
f   Posterior belly of digastric
g   Hypoglossal nerve
h   Vagus nerve
i   Glossopharyngeal nerve

For each of the anatomical descriptions below, select the single most likely structure from the options listed above. Each option may be used once, more than once or not at all.

1. This muscle crosses the carotid artery superiorly.

2. This vein crosses the carotid bifurcation.

3. This nerve crosses the external carotid artery 1 cm superior to the carotid bifurcation.

Question 10: Answers

1 – f

'Digastric' means 'two bellies'. The anterior belly runs from the mandible to the hyoid bone and is supplied by the **mandibular trigeminal** nerve (via a branch of nerve to mylohyoid). The posterior belly runs from the hyoid bone to the mastoid process and is supplied by the **facial** nerve.

2 – a

The facial vein is alongside the facial artery as the arteries cross over the body of the mandible. It drains into the internal jugular vein.

3 – g

This is an important landmark for the hypoglossal nerve as it can be easily damaged during this operation.

System Module C: Head, Neck, Endocrine and Paediatric

Questions

1	Respiratory tract	157
2	Salivary glands	159
3	Sites of upper aerodigestive tract obstruction	161
4	Lumps in the neck	163
5	Complications of thyroid surgery	165
6	Epistaxis	167
7	Adrenal pathophysiology	169
8	Paediatric constipation	171
9	Abdominal conditions in children	173
10	Paediatric urogenital conditions	175

Question 1:
Theme: Respiratory tract

Options:
- a Lower motor neurone disease
- b Glottic laryngeal carcinoma
- c Supraglottic laryngeal carcinoma
- d Subglottic laryngeal carcinoma
- e Foreign body
- f Recurrent laryngeal nerve palsy
- g Epiglottitis
- h Quinsy
- i Croup

For each of the patients described below, select the single most likely diagnosis from the options listed above. Each option may be used once, more than once or not at all.

1. A 5-year-old boy presents to the Accident and Emergency Department with severe difficulty in breathing and stridor. He appears cyanosed and is drooling. He is distressed and when he tries to speak he sounds as though he has a hot potato in his mouth.

2. A 62-year-old smoker becomes progressively more dyspnoeic over 2 months. It is possible to palpate unilateral supraclavicular lymph nodes.

3. A 65-year-old ex-smoker is noted to have clubbing.

4. A 60-year-old smoker presents with progressive inspiratory **and** expiratory stridor.

Question 1: Answers

1 – g

Epiglottitis is a potentially fatal condition. *Haemophilus influenzae* type B is the commonest pathogen. The child is often in the 'sniffing fresh air' position, with the neck extended. An anaesthetist must be called immediately as most require intubation for 1–3 days. If no anaesthetist is present, tracheostomy must be seriously considered.

2 – c

Laryngeal carcinomas are categorized by their relation to the glottis. The glottis is the area between the vocal cords (rima glottidis). Each type presents in a different way.

- **Glottic** carcinomas are the commonest (70% of laryngeal carcinomas). These arise from the vocal cords and present early as they produce hoarseness. They therefore have a favourable prognosis.

- **Supraglottic** carcinomas are the next commonest (20%). These arise from above the vocal cords, producing discomfort initially. Pain and hoarseness are late symptoms, and cervical node spread has usually occurred by the time of presentation. They have a worse prognosis. Lymph drains to the **superior** cervical lymph nodes.

- **Subglottic** carcinomas (10%) arise beneath the vocal cords. The tumour grows silently until the patient suffers hoarseness and dyspnoea. Lymph drains to the **inferior** cervical and **mediastinal** lymph nodes and helps distinguish these tumours from supraglottic tumours.

Refer to page 40.

3 – f

Clubbing has many causes, but one must always be aware of lung cancer being the potential cause, and here it is the **single most likely** cause. Lung cancer can present as a recurrent laryngeal nerve palsy either from the primary tumour or from lymph nodes. (Exam questions may ask you to think laterally in this way.)

4 – d

Inspiratory stridor is due to a narrowing of the larynx. Expiratory stridor is due to a narrowing in the bronchial tree. Inspiratory and expiratory stridor will therefore be due to a narrowing in between these areas. The only possible answer from the selection is a subglottic carcinoma.

Question 2:
Theme: Salivary glands

Options:
    a   Parotid gland
    b   Submandibular gland
    c   Sublingual gland

For each of the characteristics described below, select the single most likely salivary gland from the options listed above. Each option may be used once, more than once or not at all.

1. Its stones are the most radio-opaque.

2. Its stones are the most radiolucent.

3. Its tumours are more likely to be malignant.

4. Its secretions are the most mucinous.

5. It swells in mumps.

Question 2: Answers

1 – c

2 – a

3 – c

4 – c

5 – a

Radiolucent stones	⟶	Radio-opaque stones
Serous secretions	⟶	Mucinous secretions
Most tumours	⟶	Least tumours
Benign potential	⟶	Malignant potential

Parotid gland   Submandibular gland   Sublingual gland

If we added lacrimal glands to the question, though they are not technically a salivary gland, it is worth noting that the only disorder to affect all four glands is Sjögren's syndrome.

Question 3:
Theme: Sites of upper aerodigestive tract obstruction

Options:

    a Oropharyngeal isthmus
    b Valleculae
    c Piriform fossae
    d Cricopharyngeus
    e Thoracic inlet
    f Left main bronchus
    g Beside aortic arch
    h Beside left atrium
    i Diaphragmatic inlet
    j Gastro-oesophageal junction
    k None of the above

For each of the descriptions below, select the single most likely site of obstruction from the options listed above. Each option may be used once, more than once or not at all.

1. C6.

2. T10.

3. Fish bone.

4. 50 pence piece.

5. Peanut.

Question 3: Answers

1 – d

2 – i

3 – a

Although the piriform fossa is an often-quoted site where food gets stuck, fish bones usually get lodged in the tonsils.

4 – d

Smaller coins usually pass through the digestive tract. It is worth doing a chest X-ray (only) to show if a coin is in the oesophagus because if an object gets past the gastro-oesophageal junction, it is going to pass all the way through the digestive tract. Thus, an abdominal X-ray is pointless.

In adults, the vertebral bodies and mediastinal structures superimposed over the oesophagus are more radiodense. It may thus be necessary to do a lateral thoracic X-ray to visualize the foreign object.

5 – k

A peanut classically gets stuck in the right main bronchus, which is a straighter and wider branch of the carina, and therefore a more direct path to follow.

Food may become stuck in the digestive tract at any of the following structures, listed here in descending order with their vertebral levels:

- a – Oropharyngeal isthmus – C2 (think of a peg view X-ray)
- b – Valleculae – C4
- c – Piriform fossae – C4–5
- d – Cricopharyngeus – C6
- e – Thoracic inlet – T1
- f – Behind the left main bronchus – T4–5
- g – Behind the aortic arch – T4
- h – Behind the left atrium – T5
- i – Diaphragmatic inlet – T10
- j – Gastro-oesophageal junction – T11

Note that obstruction of the oesophagus by a left atrium that is hypertrophied from mitral stenosis is vanishingly rare (it is known as Ortner's syndrome). We know of no one who has seen a case.

Question 4:
Theme: Lumps in the neck

Options:

    a   Chemodectoma
    b   Branchial cyst
    c   Hodgkin's lymphoma
    d   Cystic hygroma
    e   Thyroglossal cyst
    f   Pharyngeal pouch
    g   Dermoid cyst
    h   Goitre
    i   Collar stud abscess

For each of the characteristics described below, select the single most likely lump from the options listed above. Each option may be used once, more than once or not at all.

1. A 20-year-old woman has a painless swelling in the upper left side of her neck. On examination it lies anterior to the upper part of her sternocleidomastoid. It is ovoid, fluctuant, with a smooth and distinct edge. There is no cervical lymphadenopathy, and she is otherwise well.

2. A 61-year-old Indian man complains of a painful lump in the upper right side of his neck. He has been feeling generally unwell, with fevers and loss of appetite. On examination, there is a 3 cm well-defined fluctuant lump partly underneath sternocleidomastoid, whose overlying skin is red-purple in colour. Despite its colour the lump is not hot.

3. A 20-year-old man presents with a painless lump in his neck. It is in the midline, rubbery hard with a smooth well-defined edge and is 2 cm in diameter. It moves up when he pokes his tongue out.

Question 4: Answers

1 – b

2 – i

3 – e

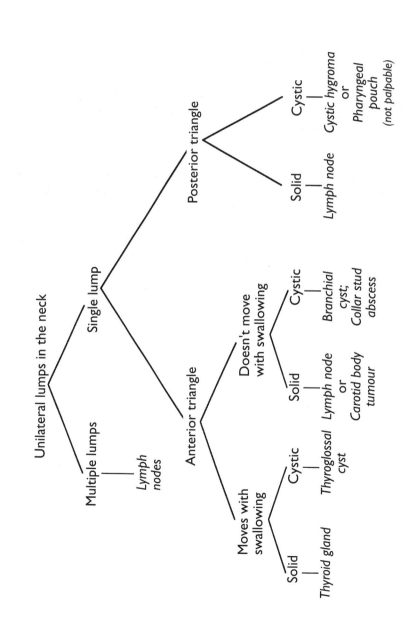

Question 5:
Theme: Complications of thyroid surgery

Options:

    a   Recurrent laryngeal nerve palsy
    b   External laryngeal nerve palsy
    c   Hypocalcaemia
    d   Hypercalcaemia
    e   Hypothyroidism
    f   Tracheomalacia
    g   Wound haemorrhage

For each of the clinical scenarios described below, select the single most likely complication from the options listed above. Each option may be used once, more than once or not at all.

1. A 51-year-old woman undergoes a total thyroidectomy for a large multinodular goitre. At the follow-up clinic she complains that she has been feeling lethargic and listless.

2. A 56-year-old woman has a generalized fit 4 days after a total thyroidectomy. She has no previous history of epilepsy.

3. A patient complains of dyspnoea after her subtotal thyroidectomy.

Question 5: Answers

1 – e

Of postoperative hypothyroidism, 90% occurs within the first year. If the patient is clinically euthyroid with a low T_4, no treatment is needed other than careful review as thyroid function may return to normal in 6–12 months. If **clinical** hypothyroidism is confirmed, it is treated with thyroxine for life.

Postoperative thyrotoxic crisis occurs if the patient has not been made medically euthyroid pre-operatively.

2 – c

Postoperative hypocalcaemia is due to parathyroid insufficiency. This may be due to removal or infarction of these glands, and usually presents 2–5 days after **total thyroidectomy**. It is rare due to meticulous surgery and routine postoperative measurement of Ca^{2+} levels.

3 – g

A **subtotal thyroidectomy** is more likely to produce wound haemorrhage as it leaves cut surfaces of the thyroid gland, which are prone to oozing. Meticulous apposition of the cut edges of the gland with purse string sutures is vital if this complication is to be avoided.

This operation is performed on the anterior part of the gland, thus avoiding the posteriorly located laryngeal nerves and parathyroid glands.

Question 6:
Theme: Epistaxis

Options:

    a   Pinch cartilagenous part of nose
    b   Tip head back
    c   Cauterize
    d   Packing
    e   Ligate external carotid artery
    f   Ligate internal carotid artery

For each of the clinical vignettes described below, select the single most likely management from the options listed above. Each option may be used once, more than once or not at all.

1. A 74-year-old man presents with a profuse nosebleed. There is no history of trauma. On examination the bleeding point appears to be coming from the posterior part of the nasal cavity.

2. A 28-year-old haemophiliac man presents with a severe nosebleed. On examination he is tachycardic with a blood pressure of 100/78 mmHg. He had his nose packed, but it continued to exsanguinate. He was therefore transferred to theatre where his ethmoidal arteries and then maxillary artery was ligated. However, he continues to bleed.

3. A patient presents to the Accident and Emergency Department and you note that he is bleeding from Kisselbach's plexus.

Question 6: Answers

1 – d

2 – e

3 – a

When a patient presents with epistaxis, assess ABC.

Epistaxis can kill. If necessary, fluid resuscitate. (A history is vital in case of a bleeding disorder.)

If not exsanguinating, sit the patient slightly forwards and ask them to press firmly against the entire cartilagenous part of the nose up to the bridge (most patients just press the tip).

If this has not stemmed blood flow in 10 min, look for the site of bleeding.

An anterior bleed is commonly from Little's area, and will therefore be a capillary bleed. It is commonly caused by trauma, and can usually be stopped by cautery. If not, an anterior pack should be adequate.

A posterior bleed is arterial and classically secondary to atherosclerosis. This is more difficult to control and will require admission with a posterior nasal pack and/or a balloon catheter.

Continuous bleeding despite these measures will require surgery.

- Repack in theatre
- Septal surgery (for deviation)
- Arterial ligation:
  - Anterior ethmoidal (branch of the internal carotid) artery
  - Maxillary (branch of the external carotid) artery – difficult
  - External carotid artery if these measures fail – easier

Question 7:
Theme: Adrenal pathophysiology

Options:
- a   Cushing's disease
- b   Cushing's syndrome
- c   Phaeochromocytoma
- d   Conn's syndrome
- e   Addison's disease
- f   Multiple endocrine neoplasia type I (Werner's syndrome)
- g   Multiple endocrine neoplasia type IIa

For each of the clinical scenarios described below, select the single most likely diagnosis from the options listed above. Each option may be used once, more than once or not at all.

1. A 60-year-old lifelong smoker presents with a history of polydipsia and polyuria. On examination, you note that he has a round face, acne, abdominal striae and hypertension.

2. A 30-year-old woman with known pernicious anaemia feels faint and weak. Investigations reveal a low blood pressure and high serum potassium concentration.

3. A 40-year-old woman presents with epigastric pain. She has a history of duodenal ulcers and hirsutism, and notes that her legs always get swollen and retain fluid. Investigations reveal hypercalcaemia.

Question 7: Answers

1 – b

This woman has an ACTH-secreting lung tumour, producing adrenal cortical hyperplasia and Cushing's syndrome. This is distinct from Cushing's **disease**, which is due to hypersecretion of ACTH from the anterior pituitary gland.

Three steps to diagnosis of Cushing's syndrome:

- A low-dose dexamethasone suppression test is performed. In a normal patient injection suppresses ACTH production, with resultant decreased cortisol levels. If levels do not decrease then the patient has Cushing's syndrome.
- A high-dose dexamethasone suppression test is performed. If cortisol levels are suppressed the source is the pituitary gland. If cortisol levels are not suppressed then the source is an adrenal tumour or an ectopic source of ACTH, e.g. lung cancer.
- Measure ACTH levels. If low, then the source of steroids is from an adrenal tumour. If high, then the source of steroids is from either the pituitary gland or an ectopic source.

2 – e

Addison's disease is adrenocortical insufficiency. Of cases, 60% is autoimmune in nature, often associated with other autoimmune conditions such as pernicious anaemia and Hashimoto's thyroiditis. Other causes are tuberculosis, metastases (lung cancer) and amyloidosis.

3 – f

Multiple endocrine neoplasia is due to neoplasia of APUD cells (**a**mine **p**recursor **u**ptake and **d**ecarboxylation). Inheritance may be sporadic or autosomal dominant. There are three types:

- MEN I – **p**arathyroid gland, **p**ancreatic islet cells and **p**ituitary gland (common). Thyroid and adrenal cortex (rarely)
- MEN IIa – parathyroid hyperplasia, medullary thyroid carcinoma, phaechromocytoma
- MEN IIb – MEN IIa + neurofibromatosis

This woman, with MEN I, could have had duodenal ulcers due to:

- Hypercalcaemia from hyperparathyroidism
- Excess steroid production from her Cushing's disease
- Zollinger–Ellinson syndrome

Question 8:
Theme: Paediatric constipation

Options:

    a   Imperforate anus
    b   Meconium ileus
    c   Hirschsprung's disease
    d   Anal fissure
    e   Rectovaginal fistula
    f   Duodenal atresia
    g   Tracheo-oesophageal fistula
    h   Ladd's bands

For each of the clinical scenarios described below, select the single most likely diagnosis from the options listed above. Each option may be used once, more than once or not at all.

1. A mother presents her 3-day-old baby to her general practitioner. She states that the baby is becoming progressively more irritable, is off its feeds and is crying continuously. Today, the baby started vomiting bilious-green liquid. The mother notes that the baby only passed its meconium yesterday, although it is passing urine freely. Examination reveals an abdomen distended by gas and faeces, a flared costal margin and the umbilicus is displaced downwards.

2. A Caucasian woman gives birth to a baby 4 weeks prematurely, which is still small for dates. She had suffered from polyhydramnios during the pregnancy. The child did not pass meconium after the birth and suffered from constipation, bilious vomiting and abdominal distension. Examination revealed thickened loops of distended bowel, but an X-ray was difficult to interpret though it had a few fluid levels. A gastrograffin enema was performed that showed defective filling in the terminal ileum. The baby improved immediately after the enema and all signs and symptoms disappeared.

3. A baby with Down's syndrome is readmitted 1 day after birth for vomiting and abdominal distension. There appears to be upper abdominal distension. An X-ray shows a 'double-bubble' of gas.

Question 8: Answers

1 – c

Hirschsprung's disease occurs in 1:4500 births, accounting for 10% of neonatal obstruction. It is caused by failure of ganglion cells migrating to the submucosa and myenteric plexus of the large bowel. The affected section is tonically contracted and aperistaltic causing the delay in passing meconium and symptoms of this case. Of babies, 95% present within a year (85% in 1 month) and an older child would have suffered intermittent bouts of constipation.

Enterocolitis with perforation and septicaemia is a complication. Per rectum examination may release meconium and air explosively. Diagnosis is confirmed by a narrowed section with proximal dilatation on barium enema, rectal biopsy (80% involve rectosigmoid) and anorectal manometry. Cure is surgical, pulling normal proximal bowel to the anus.

2 – b

Meconium ileus is associated in 5–10% with cystic fibrosis where viscid secretions obstruct the bowel. Vomiting of green rather than yellow vomit suggests a mechanical obstruction. An X-ray is often unhelpful, but is said to show 'ground-glass' bowel with fluid levels. If gastrograffin does not break up the meconium plug, ileostomy may be needed. Meconium ileus is also possibly related to early feeding with reconstituted milk, especially in the premature or low birth weight baby. They may also be cured by manual evacuation.

3 – f

Duodenal atresia produces the same signs and symptoms as an annular pancreas. (In the foetus, the duodenum is surrounded by the pancreas' ventral and dorsal parts, which fuse as the gut rotates to form the head and uncinate process.) The former, but not annular pancreas, is associated with Down's syndrome. The diagnostic 'double-bubble' is formed by air trapped in the caudal second part of the duodenum and the fundus of the stomach.

Imperforate anus will be easily seen, but if there is a fistula it is important to check the urine for meconium. In a female, a rectovaginal fistula may present much later, as all one will see is a messy perineum as the vagina acts as an outlet for faeces. An X-ray with the baby upside down will cause an air bubble to rise to the distal end of the rectum/anus and allow one to see the distance to the perineum. One can then decide whether a simple perineal incision is needed for cure, or if a colostomy and anastomosis is needed if the agenesis extends more proximally.

Ladd's bands are due to failure of caecal descent and is due to abnormal rotation in the foetus, leaving the caecum in front of the duodenum and peritoneal bands (Ladd's) twist the two parts of gut together causing obstruction. It may not present until days or weeks after birth. Volvulus neonatorum or sigmoid volvulus has a similar aetiology.

Congenital abnormalities are commonly associated with others. In this case, remember **VATER**:

- **V**ertebral
- **A**norectal
- **T**racheo-
- **E**sophageal (American spelling)
- **R**enal

Question 9:
Theme: Abdominal conditions in children

Options:

    a   Intussusception
    b   Mesenteric adenitis
    c   Meckel's diverticulum
    d   Appendicitis
    e   Strangulated inguinal hernia
    f   Hypertrophic pyloric stenosis
    g   Constipation
    h   Nephroblastoma
    i   Riedel's lobe of liver

For each of the clinical scenarios described below, select the single most likely diagnosis from the options listed above. Each option may be used once, more than once or not at all.

1. A 4-year-old boy is brought into hospital by his mother. For the past 2 days he has had a cold where he has been complaining of a sore throat, headache and nausea. Today he has vomited twice, is not keeping fluids down and complains of central abdominal pain causing him to draw his knees up to his chest. On examination he is apyrexial (but he had a temperature of 38.5°C yesterday), has a heart rate – 100 beats min^{-1} and is well hydrated. His tonsils are enlarged with no pus, eardrums both bulging and his abdomen is tender but soft.

2. A 2-year-old girl is referred urgently to clinic having presented to her general practitioner with haematuria on two occasions last week, and an abdominal mass. She is now asymptomatic. There is a firm mass with a poorly defined smooth lower border in the left upper quadrant of her abdomen. It is non-tender and not dull to percussion.

3. A 14-year-old girl complains of abdominal pain for 2 weeks, which has worsened acutely today. History reveals bright red blood loss per rectum with defecation, which she notes on the toilet paper. Her abdomen is soft with normal bowel sounds, and per rectum exam is too tender to perform, though you note an anal fissure at 6 o'clock.

4. A 1-year-old child has been noted to have bouts of screaming where he is doubled-up in agony from abdominal pain with a 60-min pain-free period in between. When you ask to see his nappy, you note a redcurrant jelly stool, with a trace of blood on his anus.

Question 9: Answers

1 – b
The child with appendicitis is usually quiet with facial flushing. Enlarged head and neck lymph nodes on examination with a history of a cold points towards mesenteric adenitis. The pyrexia is usually higher and ends quickly with mesenteric adenitis. Unfortunately (for diagnostic purposes) appendicitis has few signs of peritonism in the early stages. The longer history of this case suggests mesenteric adenitis being the **single most likely** diagnosis. Careful discussion with the parents to observe for worsening, despite analgesics and fluids, will help a diagnosis of appendicitis not being missed.

2 – h
Arising from embryological renal tissue, nephroblastomas invade locally, and metastasize to liver, lungs and bone as well as to regional nodes. The child is usually < 3 years old. Haematuria is a rare presentation (as is anorexia, weight loss, hypertension), but always bear in mind nephroblastoma with pyrexia of unknown origin. Differential diagnoses include splenomegaly (dull to percussion), hydronephrosis and post-traumatic pancreatic pseudocyst.

3 – g
A classic spiral into constipation is caused by a hard stool tearing anal mucosa to form a fissure. This makes defecation even more tender, causing the child to avoid defecation, thus worsening the constipation. Treatment of anal fissure includes dietary improvement first with fruit, vegetables and plenty of fluids, and with topical local anaesthetic (such as anusol). GTN cream is now used temporarily to relax the anal sphincter for a period long enough to allow for recovery. An anal stretch (which temporarily paralyses the external sphincter, but has a small risk of incontinence) and lateral sphincterotomy to relax the sphincter are for resistant cases.

Constipation may also be caused by a change in milk preparation, hypothyroidism, idiopathic hypercalcemia and neuromuscular disorders.

Hamartomatous polyps are the commonest cause of painless rectal bleeding in children. One must exclude familial adenomatous polyposis.

4 – a
Intussusception is an invagination of a segment of bowel (intussusceptum) into the part immediately distal to it (intussuscipiens). Peristalsis lengthens the invaginated portion and each peristaltic wave accounts for a bout of colic. It is probably due to a viral illness enlarging a Peyer's patch (in an adult, a polyp or tumour may rarely cause intussusception). A 'redcurrant stool' and sausage-shaped mass felt in the abdomen over the affected area are diagnostic; ileocaecal intussusception is the most common site. Later, the child will vomit due to the obstruction. If symptoms persist for 10 h venous infarction may occur. Urgent barium enema will confirm the diagnosis, and the hydrostatic pressure produced by lifting the bag of contrast **usually** reduces the intussusception. If not, urgent laparotomy is indicated for reduction with or without resection, depending on the viability of bowel.

Question 10:
Theme: Paediatric urogenital conditions

Options:

    a   Non-communicating hydrocoele
    b   Communicating hydrocoele
    c   Inguinal hernia
    d   Posterior urethral valves
    e   Hydrocoele of cord
    f   Phimosis
    g   Epispadias
    h   Hypospadias

For each of the clinical scenarios described below, select the single most likely diagnosis from the options listed above. Each option may be used once, more than once or not at all.

1. The mother of a newborn baby boy notices that he does not appear to be urinating from the end of his penis, and that the urinary stream points downwards. On examination his external urethral meatus is situated on the ventral aspect of his penile shaft.

2. A worried mother asks you to see her 2-year-old son as she notices that his scrotum swells up during the day and becomes smaller at night. On examination there is a fluctuant transilluminable swelling in the right scrotum which is impossible to get above. Bowel is neither felt nor heard in the swelling.

Question 10: Answers

1 – h

Hypospadias is a common congenital abnormality in which the external urethral meatus is found on the **ventral** aspect of the penis, unlike epispadias (much less common) where the meatus is on the **dorsal** side of the penis. The remainder of the urethra, distal to the meatus, becomes fibrotic causing downward bending of the penis. This is known as chordee.

The foreskin is **hooded** in appearance due to its absence on the ventral side of the penis.

2 – b

The testis descends from the posterior wall of the abdomen into the scrotum via the inguinal canal. It carries a pouch of peritoneum with it, called the **processus vaginalis**. In the first year of life the processus vaginalis becomes obliterated, leaving the tunica vaginalis surrounding the testis. If this does not happen, the scrotal sac fills with peritoneal fluid via a **communicating hydrocoele**. Because it is continuous with the peritoneal cavity, the swelling will increase on standing and decrease when lying down. If it fills with bowel, an inguinal hernia is present.

A **non-communicating hydrocoele** occurs when the processus vaginalis has closed, but re-absorption of fluid from the tunica vaginalis is incomplete. These present at birth and do not vary in size. If they have not resolved within 4–6 months of birth, the fluid may be aspirated.

System Module D: Abdomen

Questions

1	Hernia anatomy	179
2	Abdominal incisions	181
3	Abdominal stomas	185
4	Dysphagia	189
5	Acute abdominal pain	191
6	Haematemesis	193
7	Abdominal masses	195
8	Mass in the right iliac fossa	197
9	Rectal bleeding	199
10	Hepatobiliary system	201

Question 1:
Theme: Hernia anatomy

Options:

    a   Indirect inguinal hernia
    b   Direct inguinal hernia
    c   Obturator hernia
    d   Spighelian hernia
    e   Femoral hernia
    f   Epigastric hernia
    g   *Para*-umbilical hernia
    h   Umbilical hernia

For each of the anatomical locations below, select the single most likely hernia from the options listed above. Each option may be used once, more than once or not at all.

1. Emerging above and medial to the pubic tubercle and descending into the scrotum.

2. Emerging below and lateral to the pubic tubercle.

3. Emerging from the umbilicus in an adult.

4. Emerging in the upper inner thigh.

Question I: Answers

1 – a

A hernia is an abnormal protrusion of all or part of a viscus through its containing wall. Indirect inguinal hernias follow the inguinal canal from the deep ring (mid-point of the inguinal ligament) to the superficial ring (just above and medial to the pubic tubercle). It may descend from here into the scrotum.

A direct inguinal hernia is also felt through the superficial ring. As it is a protrusion through a weakened posterior wall of the inguinal canal, it protrudes anteriorly and does not classically descend into the scrotum.

A common mistake is to confuse the mid-inguinal point with the mid-point of the inguinal canal.

- The **mid-inguinal point** is half way between the anterior superior iliac spine (ASIS) and the pubic *symphisis*. It is the surface marking for the **femoral artery**
- The **mid-point of the inguinal ligament** is half way between the ASIS and the pubic *tubercle*. It is the surface marking for the **deep inguinal ring**

2 – e

Femoral herniae pass through the femoral canal, which is below and lateral to the pubic tubercle. The femoral canal is medial to the femoral vein and contains fat and lymphatics, including Cloquet's node – an important differential diagnosis of a lump in the groin. The femoral nerve is lateral to the femoral artery, which in turn is lateral to the femoral vein. This can easily be remembered by the mnemonic **NAVY** (nerve, artery, vein, Y-fronts). See page 142.

3 – g

Umbilical herniae may be congenital or acquired. Congenital herniae are always **true** umbilical herniae, i.e. they protrude through the weak scar tissue that forms when the umbilical vessels atrophy after birth. They usually close spontaneously by 2 years of age.

Acquired umbilical herniae in adults are rare, but they occur by the same mechanism. It is usually due to increased intra-abdominal pressure. Much more common is a *para*-umbilical hernia in which the protruding sac pushes the umbilicus to one side, making it a crescent-shaped slit.

4 – c

Obturator herniae protrude through the obturator foramen, which is the space between the superior pubic ramus, anterior acetabular wall and ischiopubic ramus. They commonly present as a painless lump felt in the upper inner thigh. By irritating the obturator nerve, they may also give rise to knee pain or an area of numbness in the inner thigh.

Question 2:
Theme: Abdominal incisions

Options:

    a   Thoraco-abdominal incision
    b   Milwaukee incision
    c   Midline incision
    d   Kocher incision
    e   Paramedian incision
    f   Transverse incision
    g   Gridiron incision
    h   Pfannenstiel incision

From the operations below, name the correct incision from the options listed above. Each option may be used once, more than once or not at all.

1. Elective cholecystectomy.

2. Elective right hemicolectomy.

3. Radical prostatectomy.

4. Emergency appendicectomy.

5. Emergency abdominal aortic aneurysm repair.

Question 2: Answers

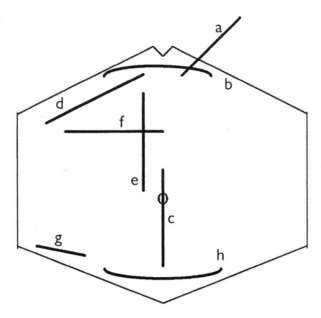

The letters above correspond to the incisions in the list of options.

Question 2: Answers

1 – d
An incision through the rectus abdominis is a muscle-**cutting** incision.
It takes more time to open and close, as this is done in layers. It is there-
fore associated with more blood loss than midline incisions.

2 – c
Midline incisions cut through the linea alba, thus avoiding any muscle
(including pyramidalis). They are therefore rapid, easily extended, quick
to close (single-layer mass technique) and associated with very little
blood loss. **Any** abdominal operation can be performed through an
extended midline incision and is thus used in emergency situations.

Paramedian incisions are reported to have lower rates of incisional
herniae (which will be your answer in the exam!). However, these
incisions are made in elective surgery on relatively well patients, which
may explain this statistic.

3 – h
The Pfannenstiel incision provides good access to the pelvis and its
organs, which lie **under** the peritoneum. It is therefore useful for lower
section Caesarean sections and radical prostatectomy. 'Pfannenstiel' is
German for frying pan handle, but the incision was named after Dr
Pfannenstiel who invented the technique.

4 – g
Made immediately medial to the anterior superior iliac spine, the
Gridiron is a muscle **splitting** incision. Currently it is more common to
use a Lanz incision, which follows a Langer's line and is therefore more
cosmetically acceptable. Both incisions involve teasing apart the muscle
fibres of the anterior abdominal wall rather than cutting through them.
Muscle-splitting incisions are purported to cause less postoperative pain
than muscle-cutting incisions.

5 – c
Note that there is no need to close the peritoneum in a midline incision.

Question 3:
Theme: Abdominal stomas

Options:
  a   Caecostomy
  b   Hartmann's procedure
  c   Loop transverse colostomy
  d   End colostomy
  e   Double-barrelled colostomy
  f   Ileostomy

For each of the clinical vignettes below, select the single most likely stoma from the options listed above. Each option may be used once, more than once or not at all.

1. A 60-year-old man presents acutely with large bowel obstruction. At laparotomy he has a neoplastic lesion in his sigmoid colon.

2. A 44-year-old woman with a long history of ulcerative colitis presented with weight loss and anaemia. In hospital she has had 1 week of bloody diarrhoea that has not responded to medical therapy. Her mother also suffered from ulcerative colitis and died of colonic carcinoma.

3. A 54-year-old man is on the list for an elective anterior resection. The operation was technically difficult with a low anastomosis and a decision is made to 'rest the bowel'.

4. You are asked to see a 70-year-old nun on the care of the elderly ward. She has not passed a stool for 6 days, which is not uncommon for her and explains her use of senna for the past 24 years. However, she has been complaining of a distended abdomen for the past 2 days. Abdominal X-ray reveals a single grossly dilated loop of sigmoid colon reaching the xiphisternum, which was not unlike a coffee bean in appearance. A flatus tube fails to resolve the situation. At laparotomy the sigmoid colon was viable.

Question 3: Answers

The diagram shows the indications for diverting the faecal stream through the anterior abdominal wall via a stoma.

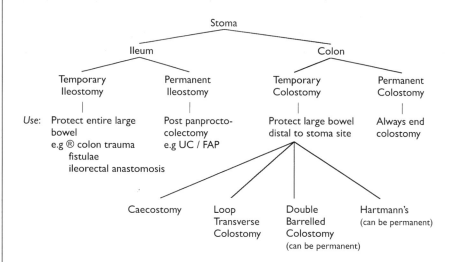

1 – b
Hartmann's procedure brings an end colostomy to the left iliac fossa, with the distal stump oversewn to allow reconnection at a later date. This is why it is used in emergency surgery where primary anastomosis is inadvisable because of obstruction, faecal contamination, inflammation or in frail and debilitated patients.

2 – f
In an **ileostomy** the bowel wall is fashioned into a spout. This is to prevent the more irritant small bowel effluent from coming into contact with the skin.

3 – c
Faeces from a **loop transverse colostomy** are much less irritant than that of an enzyme-rich ileostomy effluent. No spout is needed, and the stoma is flush with skin.

4 – e
Double-barrelled colostomies are used to defunction distal bowel. Unlike loop colostomies they avoid the risk of intestinal contents spilling into the efferent loop. This is because they are made by transecting the

bowel to form two separate limbs, which are brought out of the bowel wall together **side by side**. They can therefore be left *in situ* for longer than a loop colostomy. They can be used to replace a Hartmann's operation only when both limbs of the stoma are sufficiently long enough (8–10 cm) to be brought to the skin surface. Hence, their use in sigmoid volvulus surgery or management of sigmoid perforation (but not more distal perforation).

Caecostomies are used for peri-operative colonic lavage in unprepared obstructed colon (using a large-bore Foley catheter) before resection of the obstructing lesion and primary anastomosis. They do not decompress the bowel or protect an anastomosis efficiently, and are therefore rarely used in these circumstances any more.

Question 4:
Theme: Dysphagia

Options:

    a   Pharyngeal pouch
    b   Oesophageal carcinoma
    c   Inflammatory stricture
    d   Achalasia
    e   Plummer–Vinson syndrome
    f   Bulbar palsy
    g   Retrosternal goitre

For each of the patients below, select the single most likely pathology from the options listed above. Each option may be used once, more than once or not at all.

1. A 74-year-old smoker presents to clinic having had a 4-month history of difficulty swallowing his Sunday steak – despite his wife cutting it up into progressively smaller pieces for him. He is now finding it increasingly difficult to swallow his porridge in the morning. His general practitioner referral letter indicates no past history of dyspepsia.

2. A 35-year-old man presents to casualty with a productive cough and pyrexia. His coughing usually occurs at night. Detailed questioning reveals that he has had difficulty in swallowing fluids. Recently, he has noticed some retrosternal pain.

3. A 52-year-old trainspotter with halitosis presents to his general practitioner with a history of recurrent sore throats. He is sent home on antibiotics, but this does not resolve the problem. He now presents to the Accident and Emergency Department having noticed a lump on the left side of his neck.

Question 4: Answers

1 – b
It is important to remember that oesophageal carcinoma can present **de novo** as in this case, or secondary to other oesophageal disorders such as peptic oesophagitis (Barrett's oesophagus), achalasia or a pharyngeal pouch.

2 – d
Achalasia is believed to be a failure of the oesophageal sphincter to relax due to a defect of the parasympathetic Auerbach's myenteric plexus. It is unusual in that patients often present with difficulty swallowing **fluids** ± solids. The patient eats slowly and may even use the Valsalva manoeuvre to force food from the oesophagus into the stomach. Regurgitation from the dilated oesophagus may cause aspiration pneumonia.

Bulbar palsy is due to damage to cranial nerves IX, X and XII. Patients will have the signs and symptoms of dysfunction of these nerves and commonly have nasal regurgitation of food.

3 – a
Pharyngeal pouches most commonly present with regurgitation of food and often with dysphagia – our patient had a rather rare presentation! It is due to a mucosal outpouching between the **two parts** of the inferior constrictor – thyropharyngeus above and cricopharyngeus below. This potential gap is called **Killian's dehiscence**.

Food is pushed from the pharynx above to the oesophagus below by the sequential contraction of the superior, middle and thyropharyngeus constrictors. Then the cricopharyngeus, acting as a sphincter, must relax to allow food to enter the oesophagus. If it does not relax, the pressure above will produce a **posterior** outpouching through the weak Killian's dehiscence. It can not expand posteriorly due to the adjacent vertebrae, and therefore descends down the back of the oesophagus to present as a lump in the posterior triangle of the neck. This is usually on the left as the oesophagus lies on the left side of the vertebral bodies.

Question 5:
Theme: Acute abdominal pain

Options:

a   Acute appendicitis
b   Acute cholecystitis
c   Renal colic
d   Acute pancreatitis
e   Ectopic pregnancy
f   Perforated peptic ulcer
g   Leaking abdominal aortic aneurysm
h   Torsion of ovarian cyst
i   Mesenteric infarction

For each of the emergency presentations below, select the single most likely diagnosis from the options listed above. Each option may be used once, more than once or not at all.

1. A 27-year-old woman presents with a 3-h history of extreme abdominal pain radiating to both shoulders. On examination she is sweaty, distressed, with a pale thready pulse. Her heart rate = 140 beats min⁻¹ and regular, blood pressure = 84/32 mmHg. Her abdomen is generally tender with rebound and guarding and an appendectomy scar. Pelvic examination is very uncomfortable.

2. A 32-year-old man presents to the Accident and Emergency Department with a 6-h history of severe left groin pain. He was initially going to present 3 h ago, but the pain eased off. It has now returned with a vengeance. He is haemodynamically stable and his abdomen is soft with normal bowel sounds.

3. You are asked to see a 76-year-old man on the cardiology ward. He is in atrial fibrillation and is complaining of a 4-h history of severe abdominal pain which he can not localize. During the consultation he becomes progressively more unresponsive, cold and clammy.

Question 5: Answers

1 – e

An ectopic pregnancy must be suspected in any woman of childbearing age with abdominal pain, especially if she is shocked. Make sure you do an HCG test!

2 – c

Renal colic, with its writhing pain from loin to groin, typically has severe exacerbating bouts lasting a few minutes. It is a true colicky pain just like uterine contractions during labour.

3 – i

The vague nature of this question reflects the vague presentation of this condition! It is difficult to diagnose, and therefore a high index of suspicion is needed as the paucity of signs and symptoms do not reflect the severity of the underlying time bomb.

Our patient was on the cardiology ward and was in atrial fibrillation. Did he have a recent myocardial infarction with resulting mural thrombus, or was the embolus simply due to his atrial fibrillation? In both conditions a clot may embolize to gut, blocking the **superior** mesenteric artery. This supplies the area from the second part of the duodenum to the distal third of the transverse colon.

Atherosclerotic mesenteric arteries may cause gut claudication, in which the patient suffers abdominal pain after meals. Mesenteric ischaemia may also be due to mesenteric **venous** thrombosis, or low cardiac output.

Question 6:
Theme: Haematemesis

Options:
- a   Mallory–Weiss tear
- b   Bleeding chronic peptic ulcer
- c   Oesophageal varices
- d   Carcinoma of the stomach
- e   Acute gastric erosion
- f   Haemophilia

For each of the patients below, select the single most likely cause of hae-matemesis from the options listed above. Each option may be used once, more than once or not at all.

1. A 31-year-old travel writer presents to the Accident and Emergency Department having vomited an estimated 500 ml bright red blood. On examination he has multiple spider naevi on his upper chest and appears slightly icteric.

2. A previously fit and well 71-year-old woman twisted her ankle on an uneven paving stone. She bought some ibuprofen tablets from the chemist 4 days ago and has been taking them regularly. She presents to the Accident and Emergency Department having just vomited a small amount of fresh red blood.

3. A 25-year-old man has 8 pints of beer on his best friend's wedding night. Much to his dismay he vomits up his meal and continues to retch afterwards. His fourth vomit contains bright red blood.

Question 6: Answers

1 – c

Although peptic ulceration is the commonest cause of haematemesis, this young writer has most likely picked up hepatitis B on his travels – hence the spider naevi and icterus. In the UK, cirrhosis is the most common cause of portal hypertension (causing 90% of varices), but worldwide the primary cause is hepatic fibrosis due to schistosomiasis. The backpressure of portal hypertension results in the development of enlarged collateral channels between portal and systemic veins, at the sites where these two circulations meet. These abnormal dilatations are known as varices, and are prone to bleeding.

Sites of portosystemic anastomosis are:

- Between the left gastric vein (portal) and oesophageal veins (systemic)
- Between the superior rectal vein (portal) and middle/inferior rectal veins (systemic)
- Between the obliterated umbilical vein (portal) and superior/inferior epigastric veins (systemic)
- Between veins of organs with no mesentery that are retroperitoneal (portal) and the posterior abdominal wall with which they are in contact (systemic). (Retroperitoneal organs are the ascending and descending colon, pancreas, second and third parts of the duodenum and the bare area of the liver)

2 – e

Non-steroidal anti-inflammatory drugs, steroids and alcohol are the most common cause of acute gastric erosions.

3 – a

A classic history of a Mallory–Weiss oesophageal tear.

Question 7:
Theme: Abdominal masses

Options:
-   a   Fibroid uterus
-   b   Riedel's lobe
-   c   Carcinoma of the caecum
-   d   Hepatitis B
-   e   Liver abscess
-   f   Polycystic kidneys
-   g   Acute retention of urine
-   h   Nephroblastoma (Wilm's tumour)
-   i   Intussusception
-   j   Ascending cholangitis

For each of the cases below, select the single most likely cause of their abdominal mass from the options listed above. Each option may be used once, more than once or not at all.

1. A 42-year-old banker has had nausea and decreased appetite for 1 week. He returned from Thailand 6 weeks ago. He is now complaining of upper abdominal pain and aching joints. On examination, he is jaundiced, pyrexial and sweaty, with a tender smooth mass in the right upper quadrant of his abdomen.

2. A 41-year-old man presents to the Accident and Emergency Department complaining of an excruciatingly painful left-sided headache of sudden onset while gardening 20 min ago. The pain is constant and he complains of nausea. His father recently died of a stroke. On examination he is anxious, tachycardic with a blood pressure = 186/124 with signs of meningism. On palpation of his abdomen you find bilateral loin masses, which move with respiration.

3. A 16-year-old boy attends routine medical examination on joining the Army. He is fit and well, with no past medical history. On abdominal examination there is a smooth, non-tender mass in the right upper quadrant extending towards the right loin.

4. A 40-year-old woman complains of a 12-h history of acute lumbar pain with numbness down her left leg that occurred when she was moving furniture. She now has lower abdominal pain and has not passed urine today. On examination of her abdomen she has a tender mass arising from her pelvis extending towards her umbilicus.

Question 7: Answers

1 – d

We will not ask how this man caught hepatitis B. The typical incubation period is between 1 and 6 months, as opposed to hepatitis A, which is between 2 and 6 weeks. Ascending cholangitis is a less likely diagnosis as one would expect a previous history of gallstones and it typically affects women.

2 – f

Berry aneurysms are associated with 10–30% of patients with polycystic kidneys and may cause subarachnoid haemorrhages, as in this case. Note Charcot–Bouchard micro-aneurysms (0.8–1 mm diameter) may develop secondary to the hypertension of polycystic kidneys and are more likely to produce intracerebral haemorrhage if they rupture.

Polycystic kidneys can present throughout life in many different ways:

- At birth – causing obstructed labour
- Stillbirth – often with multiple congenital abnormalities
- Incidental finding of bilateral loin masses on routine examination
- Renal failure
- Hypertension

and rarely

- Haematuria
- Loin pain
- Urinary tract infection.

3 – b

Riedel's lobe is an extended tongue-like right lobe of the liver. It is not pathological; it is a normal anatomical variant and may extend into the pelvis. It is often mistaken for a distended gallbladder or liver tumour.

4 – g

A vertebral disc may prolapse directly posteriorly (central prolapse). If this occurs it may press on the S2, 3 and 4 spinal nerves, resulting in acute urinary retention. Note that it is more common for a disc to prolapse posterolaterally as the posterior longitudinal ligament usually prevents central prolapse.

Question 8:
Theme: Mass in the right iliac fossa

Options:
  a   Iliac artery aneurysm
  b   Carcinoma of the caecum
  c   Iliac lymph node
  d   Psoas abscess
  e   Appendix mass
  f   Terminal ileitis
  g   Actinomycosis
  h   Tumour in undescended testis

For each of the cases below, select the single most likely cause of their abdominal mass from the options listed above. Each option may be used once, more than once or not at all.

1. A 15-year-old recent Indian immigrant has had malaise, night sweats and persistent backache for 1 month. Recently he has noticed a swelling in his groin, which lies below his inguinal ligament. On abdominal examination you note a swelling in the right iliac fossa, which may be emptied into the groin lump below by direct pressure.

2. A 62-year-old woman presents to her general practitioner having felt lethargic for 2 months. She has also started to become short of breath on exertion, and noticed that her wedding ring is too big for her finger. On examination she has pallor and a non-tender firm mass in the right iliac fossa.

3. A previously healthy 81-year-old woman collapses at home after suffering a bout of lower abdominal pain. Her heart rate = 140 beats min^{-1}, blood pressure = 80/30 mmHg. On examination you note a tender pulsatile mass in the right iliac fossa.

4. A 17-year-old man presents to the Accident and Emergency Department 3 weeks after an appendicectomy complaining of abdominal pain and a watery discharge from his wound site. On examination he has a thick and offensive discharge from his Lanz incision emerging from multiple sinuses. Underneath is a right iliac fossa mass.

Question 8: Answers

1 – d

This patient has a psoas abscess. It is often caused by tuberculosis of the spine (Pott's disease), which forms a paravertebral abscess that tracks down the psoas fascia overlying the muscle. The psoas muscle passes underneath the inguinal ligament and is inserted into the lesser trochanter of the femur. A psoas abscess therefore may be seen at this point in the thigh and mimic a femoral hernia. Its contents may be pushed back into the right iliac fossa, or the other way round as in our patient.

An abdominal X-ray of this patient may show a bulge in the affected psoas shadow, which would be even more obvious if the abscess was old and had calcified.

2 – b

The commonest presentation of carcinoma of the caecum is iron deficiency anaemia due to silent bleeding into the colon.

3 – a

The aorta bifurcates into the common iliac arteries, either of which may become aneurysmal and leak.

4 – g

Actinomycosis is a rare infection that examiners love asking about. These Gram-positive bacteria are commensals in the mouth and intestine. The patient is likely to be infected by *Actinomyces israelii*. Bacteriological examination of the pus reveals characteristic sulphur granules. It is treated by surgery, and 4–6 six weeks of intravenous penicillin, followed by oral penicillin for some weeks.

Question 9:
Theme: Rectal bleeding

Options:

  a   Haemorrhoids
  b   Ulcerative colitis
  c   Crohn's disease
  d   Diverticulitis
  e   Duodenal ulcer
  f   Carcinoma of the rectum
  g   Anal fissure
  h   Carcinoma of the anus

For each of the patients below, select the single most likely cause of their rectal bleeding from the options listed above. Each option may be used once, more than once or not at all.

1. A 40-year-old businessman notices that his stools have become black and tarry.

2. A 29-year-old man presents with bright red blood streaking his stool. Defecation is extremely painful, with blood on the toilet paper and in the bowl. Per rectum examination is limited due to pain, but no lump is felt.

3. A 60-year-old woman presents having passed an estimated 400 ml bright red blood per rectum and now feels faint. She has a history of chronic lower abdominal pain, flatulence, abdominal distension, belching and intermittent constipation, but has never suffered a rectal bleed. On examination she is pyrexial and sweaty with a heart rate = 110 beats min^{-1} and blood pressure = 100/55 mmHg. She is tender in the left iliac fossa, with guarding, with no masses palpable. Per rectum examination is tender on the left, with fresh blood on the glove.

4. A 64-year-old man complains of a 3-month history of intermittent diarrhoea, anorexia and weight loss. He has now had 1 week of passing painless motions with dark red blood mixed in with the stool.

Question 9: Answers

1 – e
Melaena is black due to the blood being digested by intestinal enzymes and bacteria. The bleeding must therefore arise **proximal** to the large bowel.

2 – g
A fissure-*in-ano* is a split in the anal epithelium, usually caused by trauma from passing hard stool and may become chronic if the patient has high anal sphincter tone or chronic constipation. It is usually posterior. It is acutely painful because it is a tear in the anal skin rather than the mucosa above. The former has a somatic sensory nerve supply, whereas the latter is autonomic and thus painless.

Similarly, carcinoma of the anus causes painful defecation only when the tumour is located below Hilton's white line (now called the intersphincteric groove), i.e. squamous cell carcinomas. Adenocarcinomas that arise above the intersphincteric groove are not painful unless they invade skin.

Known causes of fissure-*in-ano* include:
- Crohn's disease (multiple fissures are virtually pathognomonic of Crohn's)
- Iatrogenic (post-haemorrhoidectomy)
- STDs
- Anterior fissures may be predisposed to post-childbirth
- Chronic constipation

3 – d
The woman had the symptoms of chronic diverticular disease. An acute flare up is called diverticulitis and may be caused by stool being trapped in a diverticulum and causing inflammation. It is like 'left-sided appendicitis'.

Complications of diverticulitis include:
- Haemorrhage
- Peritonitis
- Diverticular abscess
- Intestinal obstruction
- Fistulae in 5% (vesicocolic being the commonest)

4 – f
Right-sided cancer of the colon commonly presents with anaemia ± weight loss. Transverse and left-sided colonic cancer presents with change in bowel habit, blood mixed with stool ± weight loss.

Question 10:
Theme: Hepatobiliary system

Options:

    a   ERCP and sphincterotomy
    b   Cholecystectomy with T-tube in common bile duct
    c   Laparoscopic cholecystectomy within 48 h
    d   Elective laparoscopic cholecystectomy
    e   Ursodeoxycholic acid
    f   Whipple's procedure
    g   Open cholecystectomy

For each of the patients below, select the single most likely treatment from the options listed above. Each option may be used once, more than once or not at all.

1. A 30-year-old woman with a history of von Willebrandt's disease presents with acute cholecystitis. Ultrasound scan has revealed no dilatation of the common bile duct. Liver function tests are normal.

2. A 27-year-old woman presents with pyrexia, rigors and jaundice. Liver function tests show an ALP = 480, AST = 42 and Amylase = 40. An ultrasound scan shows a dilated common bile duct.

3. A 44-year-old woman with a history of chronic cholecystitis has been shown to have a stone in the common bile duct on USS. This could not be removed at ERCP.

Question 10: Answers

1 – g

2 – a

3 – b

When thinking of biliary stone disease, remember that **jaundice** is caused only when the common bile duct (CBD) is blocked, whether due to gallstones or due to external pressure from an enlarged gallbladder.

All patients with cholecystitis should have an ultrasound scan (USS).

If the USS shows stone(s) in the gallbladder **only**, then they will **only** require cholecystectomy. This can be done either acutely, after the acute symptoms have been controlled (usually within 48 h of the attack, as an acutely inflamed gallbladder is thought to be easier to remove) or as an elective procedure. The woman in question 1 had a clotting disorder, which is an absolute contraindication to laparoscopic cholecystectomy. Other absolute contraindications are abdominal sepsis and late pregnancy. Relative contraindications include previous abdominal surgery (risk of adhesions), acute gallstone pancreatitis, untreated bile duct stones and intra-abdominal malignancy.

If the USS shows a **dilated** CBD, this suggests that a stone has passed into it from the gallbladder. If so, then the bile duct needs to be imaged either by ERCP or peri-operative cholangiogram ('on-table') and then the stone **removed**. This is because a blockage may cause ascending cholangitis, which is potentially fatal.

All patients **with** ascending cholangitis need urgent ERCP and sphincterotomy. The stone in the CBD may then be removed by a Dormia basket.

In patients **without** ascending cholangitis, the stone(s) in the CBD may be removed either at ERCP or at the time of cholecystectomy. If it is necessary to open the CBD to retrieve the stones, or stones are suspected, it is important to insert a T-tube which will drain bile percutaneously **and** allow X-ray imaging of the CBD up to 10 days after the operation.

- As a general rule, if a patient has jaundice or abnormal LFTs, then ERCP and sphincterotomy is preferred
- T-tube insertion is now primarily reserved for cases where ERCP fails to remove stones, or the CBD has been damaged.

System Module E: Urinary System and Renal Transplantation

Questions

1	Haematuria	205
2	Renal physiology	207
3	Management of renal tract calculi	209
4	Urological anatomy	211
5	Testicular conditions	213
6	Anatomy of the pelvis	215
7	Staging of bladder cancer	217
8	Renal function	219
9	Carcinoma of the prostate	221
10	Transplantation	223

Question I:
Theme: Haematuria

Options:

    a   Staghorn calculus
    b   Renal cell carcinoma
    c   Pyelonephritis
    d   Ureteric stone
    e   Transitional cell carcinoma of the bladder
    f   Schistosomiasis
    g   Carcinoma of the prostate
    h   Prostatitis
    i   March haemaglobinuria

For each of the clinical vignettes described below, select the single most likely diagnosis from the options listed above. Each option may be used once, more than once or not at all.

1. A 57-year-old man presents with a one week history of fever and pain in his left loin, with no dysuria. On examination a mass can be felt in his left loin. Urinary microscopy shows microscopic haematuria with no organisms.

2. A 24-year-old marathon runner passes blood in her urine throughout micturition shortly after beginning training for the next race. Abdominal examination and X-ray are unremarkable.

3. A 68-year-old man presents with a 2-day history of painless frank haematuria. He is worried because it happened once before 3 months ago. This morning he noticed that there were a few globular clots within the urine. On examination, his abdomen is soft and rectal examination is unremarkable.

Question I: Answers

1 – b

Renal cell carcinoma is also known as hypernephroma, Grawitz tumour or clear cell carcinoma. The classic triad of presentation occurs in 10–15% of patients:

- Loin pain
- Loin mass
- Haematuria

There are also many unusual features:

- Polycythaemia – secondary to excess erythropoetin production
- Hypercalcaemia – secondary to ectopic parathormone production by the tumour
- Cannon ball metastases – which **may** disappear after nephrectomy
- Pyrexia of unknown origin
- Nephrotic syndrome – rare

2 – i

This is not red blood cells in the urine, but **haemoglobin** from red cells that have been traumatized by severe exercise. Whether this is due to defective red cell membranes is unknown. The condition is self-limiting. Similarly, remember to ask patients with haematuria whether they had beetroot for supper, or if they are taking rifampicin. If the urine turns red on standing, investigate for porphyria.

3 – e

Transitional cell carcinoma of the bladder is the commonest cause of painless haematuria. Transitional epithelium lines the entire urinary tract, so these tumours arise from the renal pelvis to the end of the urethra in females and to the end of the prostatic urethra in males. If left untreated local invasion of a bladder neck carcinoma may cause incontinence. Obstructive hydronephrosis and clot retention are also complications.

Remember to ask for a history of foreign travel to exclude bilharzia (≡ schistosomiasis), which is the commonest cause of bladder cancer worldwide.

Question 2:
Theme: Renal physiology

Options:

     a 0.5 ml/min^{-1}
     b 11 ml/min^{-1}
     c 125 ml/min^{-1}
     d 416 ml/min^{-1}
     e 550 ml/min^{-1}
     f 909 ml/min^{-1}
     g 1111 ml/min^{-1}

For each of the calculations described below, select the single most likely answer from the options listed above. Each option may be used once, more than once or not at all.

1. Calculate glomerular filtration rate (GFR) from the following:

- Urine inulin concentration $= 37.5$ mg/ml^{-1}
- Plasma inulin concentration $= 0.3$ mg/ml^{-1}
- Volume of urine flow $= 60$ ml h^{-1}

2. Calculate the renal plasma flow (RPF) from the following:

- Urine *para*-amino hippuric acid (PAH) concentration $= 16.5$ mg/ml^{-1}
- Plasma PAH concentration $= 0.03$ mg/ml^{-1}
- Volume of urine flow $= 1$ ml/min^{-1}

3. Calculate the renal blood flow (RBF) from the following:

- Urine *para*-amino hippuric acid (PAH) concentration $= 15$ mg/ml^{-1}
- Plasma PAH concentration $= 0.03$ mg/ml^{-1}
- Volume of urine flow $= 1$ ml/min^{-1}
- Haematocrit $= 45\%$

Question 2: Answers

1 – c

2 – e

3 – f

$$GFR = \frac{\text{Urine inulin concentration } (\mathbf{U}) \times \text{volume of urine flow } (\mathbf{V})}{\text{Plasma inulin concentration } (\mathbf{P})}$$

$$RPF = \frac{\text{Urine PAH concentration } (\mathbf{U}) \times \text{volume of urine flow } (\mathbf{V})}{\text{Plasma PAH concentration } (\mathbf{P})}$$

$$RBF = \frac{RPF}{(1 - \text{haematocrit})}$$

Question 3:
Theme: Management of renal tract calculi

Options:

a   Conservative treatment (watch and wait)
b   Percutaneous nephrolithotomy (PCNL) alone
c   Extracorporeal shock wave lithotripsy (ESWL) alone
d   Percutaneous nephrostomy
e   Percutaneous nephrolithotomy followed by ESWL
f   'Push-bang' treatment
g   Dormia basket retrieval

For each of the clinical scenarios described below, select the single most likely method of management from the options listed above. Each option may be used once, more than once or not at all.

1. A 34-year-old woman presents with acute renal colic. Intravenous urogram (IVU) reveals a 0.8 cm diameter stone causing obstruction just below the right pelvi-ureteric junction of her urinary tract.

2. A 38-year-old man presents with acute renal colic. IVU reveals a 0.3 cm diameter stone midway along his left ureter with no obstruction.

3. A 29-year-old woman presents with acute renal colic. IVU reveals a 0.5 cm stone in the upper third obstructing her right ureter. She develops a fever after a few hours, and the pain becomes continuous. A subsequent IVU demonstrates that the contrast medium is not draining past the stone.

Question 3: Answers

1 – f (this is the most likely answer)

2 – a

3 – d

Management of acute renal colic:

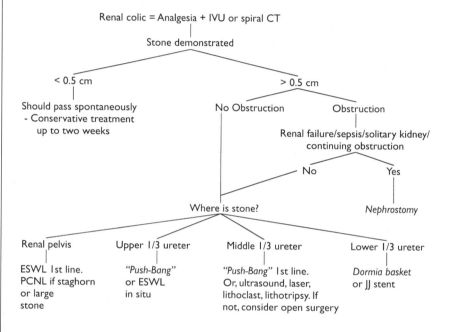

Push–Bang involves a catheter and stent pushing the stone up to the kidney for crushing by ESWL.

Open surgery has become more rare with the advent of minimally invasive procedures. It still has a place in modern urological surgery, such as when repeated ureteroscopic procedures fail.

- ESWL = extracorporeal shock wave lithotripsy
- PCNL = percutaneous nephrolithotomy

Question 4:
Theme: Urological anatomy

Options:

    a   Inferior vena cava
    b   Splenic vein
    c   Renal vein
    d   Uterine artery
    e   Internal iliac artery
    f   Superior vesical artery
    g   Deep inguinal lymph nodes
    h   Superficial inguinal lymph nodes
    i   Para-aortic lymph nodes

For each of the descriptions below, select the single most likely structure from the options listed above. Each option may be used once, more than once or not at all.

1. The only artery which crosses superior to the ureter.

2. The vein into which the right testicular vein will drain.

3. Testicular cancers will drain into these lymph nodes.

Question 4 : Answers

1 – d

The uterine artery crosses over the ureter in the female pelvis. The urine passing underneath the uterine artery gives rise to the expression 'water under the bridge'. This is an important anatomical relation because the uterine artery is tied here during a hysterectomy. It is not unheard of for the ureter to have been tied off instead!

As the ureter lies adjacent to the lateral fornix of the vagina at this point; it is interesting to note that this is the only place in the human body where it is possible to feel a ureteric stone.

2 – a

The left gonadal (i.e. testicular or ovarian) vein drains into the left renal vein, and the right gonadal vein drains directly into the inferior vena cava. Examiners love this question.

3 – i

The testicles (and ovaries) originate in the abdomen and have dragged their blood supply from the aorta. Hence, the lymphatics drain to the para-aortic lymph nodes.

Question 5:
Theme: Testicular conditions

Options:
- a   Indirect inguinal hernia
- b   Teratoma
- c   Seminoma
- d   Varicocoele
- e   Torsion of testis
- f   Torsion of hydatid of Morgagni
- g   Acute epididymo-orchitis
- h   Epididymocoele

For each of the clinical vignettes described below, select the single most likely diagnosis from the options listed above. Each option may be used once, more than once or not at all.

1. A 25-year-old man notices a hard lump on his left testicle while in the bath. Investigations reveal a positive pregnancy test.

2. A 19-year-old fireman develops sudden excruciating pain in his right testicle. There is no history of trauma. On examination, he is apyrexial and there is a small, very tender lump on the superior pole of the right testicle. The testicle appears to be in the normal position.

Question 5: Answers

1 – b

The majority of testicular tumours are either seminomas or teratomas:

	Teratoma	Seminoma
Age of patient (years)	20–30	30–40
% Testicular tumours	40	60
Substances produced	α-fetoprotein, β-HCG	LDH, β-HCG
Pathology	Variegated surface when cut	Homogenous surface when cut
Treatment sensitivity	Chemosensitive	Radiosensitive

2 – f

A cyst of the hydatid of Morgagni is also known as the appendix testis. It is the remnant of the Müllerian duct and is at the top of the testis. Its equivalent in females is the fimbriated end of the fallopian tube. It may become twisted upon itself, causing a painful lump and is similar in presentation to testicular torsion or epididymo-orchitis. For examination purposes a torted testicle will be higher and lie on its side and epididymitis will cause a pyrexia; thus, our patient could only have had a twisted appendix testis.

Question 6:
Theme: Anatomy of the pelvis

Options:

- a   Verumontanum
- b   Median lobe of the prostate
- c   Trigone
- d   Fundus of bladder
- e   Median umbilical ligament
- f   Medial umbilical ligament
- g   Lateral umbilical ligament
- h   Seminal vesicle

For each of the descriptions below, select the single most likely structure from the options listed above. Each option may be used once, more than once or not at all.

1. This is located in the bladder between the openings of the two ureters and the urethra.

2. Ablation distal to this structure during transurethral resection of prostate will result in incontinence of urine.

3. This is the remnant of the foetal urachus.

Question 6: Answers

1 – c

The trigone is a small triangle at the base of the bladder found between the internal urethral opening and the two ureters. It is a **non-distendible** part of the bladder and is rich in pain receptors.

2 – a

The prostatic urethra is kidney-shaped in cross-section. The dimple of this 'kidney' shape forms the middle of the posterior wall and is called the verumontanum. The distal urethral sphincter surrounds it. It is therefore to be avoided during transurethral surgery lest the patient is rendered incontinent.

3 – e

On the posterior aspect of the anterior abdominal wall, three ligaments are found:

- **Median umbilical ligament** – remnant of urachus
- **Medial umbilical ligament** – remnant of umbilical artery (one on each side)
- **Lateral umbilical ligament** – fold of peritoneum containing inferior epigastric vessels

Question 7:
Theme: Staging of bladder cancer

Options:

 a   Tis
 b   Ta
 c   TI
 d   T2
 e   T3a
 f   T3b
 g   T4a
 h   T4b

For each of the descriptions below, select the single most likely stage of bladder cancer from the options listed above. Each option may be used once, more than once or not at all.

1. The tumour has invaded the full thickness of the bladder wall but has not extended into the surrounding organs or pelvic wall.

2. The tumour has invaded through the bladder wall and into the prostate only.

3. The tumour has invaded into the muscle of the bladder wall but is not palpable bimanually after resection.

Question 7: Answers

1 – f

2 – g

3 – d

Stage	Depth of invasion	Treatment
Tis	Flat (non-polypoid). Not through basement membrane	Intravesical chemotherapy, e.g. BCG or antibiotics. Cystectomy if this fails
Ta	Polypoid, not through basement membrane	Transurethral resection, or biopsy and cystodiathermy + intravesical chemotherapy. Regular surveillance
T1	Penetrating basement membrane	Same as Ta unless grade is G3 – then consider cystectomy or radiotherapy
T2	Muscle in bladder wall invaded – **not** palpable bimanually post-resection	Transurethral excision of polypoid part of tumour and biopsy to stage muscle invasion. Can treat with cystectomy ± radiotherapy, and chemotherapy if preferred
T3a	Muscle invaded, tumour palpable bimanually post-resection	As for T2. Consider orthotopic bladder reconstruction or urinary diversion for all patients undergoing cystectomy
T3b	Tumour invades through full thickness of bladder wall	As for T2
T4a	Tumour invades into adjacent organs	As for T2
T4b	Tumour invades other pelvic organs or pelvic wall	Palliative radiotherapy and chemotherapy

The table has been derived from *Guidelines for the Investigation and Treatment of Urological Cancers in the United Kingdom* (London, British Association of Urological Surgeons).

Grading system for bladder cancer:

- G_1 – well differentiated
- G_2 – moderately differentiated
- G_3 – poorly or undifferentiated

Question 8:
Theme: Renal function

Options:
  a   Proximal convoluted tubule
  b   Descending limb of the loop of Henle
  c   Ascending limb of the loop of Henle
  d   Distal convoluted tubule
  e   Collecting duct

For each of the physiological processes described below, select a single most likely site of action from the options listed above. Each option may be used once, more than once, or not at all.

1. Definitive control of serum potassium concentration.

2. Glucose re-absorption.

3. Sodium re-absorption.

4. Production of a hyperosmolar medullary interstitium.

Question 8: Answers

1 – d

2 – a

3 – a

4 – c

The kidney regulates osmolarity of the body among other tasks. Each kidney takes 10% of total cardiac output and this blood is filtered in the glomerulus, allowing only molecules < 100,000 kDa to be filtered.

About two-thirds of filtered Na^+ and Cl^- ions are reabsorbed from the filtrate in the proximal convoluted tubule (PCT), leaving a hyposmolar fluid to pass to the loop of Henle.

It is then best to think of the **ascending limb** of the Loop of Henle. This is **impermeable** to water, but pumps out Na^+ ions (and Cl^- ions follow) into the renal medullary interstitium. This, therefore, provides a concentration gradient with the **descending limb** of the loop, which **is** permeable to water.

As the descending limb is being presented with **hypo**-osmolar filtrate from the PCT, it therefore gains more and more NaCl as it descends into the renal medulla, becoming **hyper**osmolar. The highest concentration of NaCl is thus at the bottom tip of the Loop of Henle, and this is what is pumped out as the filtrate passes up the ascending loop to the distal convoluted tubule, which is thus presented with a very hypotonic (water-rich) filtrate.

The distal convoluted tubule is where aldosterone acts to absorb K^+ ions, leaving only the collecting duct to 'fine tune' water absorption via the action of antidiuretic hormone (ADH).

Question 9:
Theme: Carcinoma of the prostate

Options:

    a   Hormonal manipulation
    b   Open prostatectomy and radiotherapy
    c   Palliative radiotherapy
    d   Cytotoxic chemotherapy
    e   Transurethral resection of prostate (TURP)
    f   Tamoxifen
    g   Watch and wait

For each of the patients described below, select a single most likely management from the options listed above. Each option may be used once, more than once, or not at all.

1. A 52-year-old man presents to his general practitioner with a history of rectal bleeding. While performing a rectal examination, it is noted that he has a hard lump in his prostate. Biopsy demonstrates a prostatic adenocarcinoma, which is intracapsular and surrounded by normal prostate.

2. A 71-year-old man presents with acute urinary retention. He undergoes TURP and a well-differentiated prostatic adenocarcinoma is found in four of 60 chips from the prostatectomy specimen.

3. A 80-year-old man with established carcinoma of the prostate is noted to have a non-tender wedge fracture of the fourth lumbar vertebra. He has already had a bilateral orchidectomy.

4. A 75-year-old man presents with back pain. Investigations reveal a carcinoma of the prostate, and a bone scan confirms spread to the lumbar spine.

Question 9: Answers

1 – b

2 – a

3 – g

4 – c

Stage	Degree of invasion	Treatment
T1	Intracapsular tumour surrounded by normal prostate	Radical prostatectomy or external beam radiotherapy. Hormone manipulation may be used
T2	Tumour confined to but deforming gland	As for T1
T3	Tumour beyond capsule, with lateral sulci and/or seminal vesicle invasion	Radiotherapy, hormone manipulation or both. Watch and wait if preferred
T4	Tumour fixed and invading surrounding structures	Hormone therapy with or without radiotherapy. Watch and wait if no symptoms. Radiotherapy for pain from bone metastases

We recognise that the treatment of prostatic cancer is a very controversial area. The above table has been derived from *Guidelines for the Investigation and Treatment of Urological Cancers in the United Kingdom* (London, British Association of Urological Surgeons).

Question 10:
Theme: Transplantation

Options:

    a   Renal transplant
    b   Liver transplant
    c   Heart/lung transplant
    d   Pancreas transplant
    e   Small bowel transplant
    f   Corneal transplant

For each of the descriptions below, select a single most likely transplant from the options listed above. Each option may be used once, more than once, or not at all.

1. The organ may be preserved for 18 h using the University of Wisconsin solution.

2. There is no age limit for donation of this tissue.

3. Malignancy is not necessarily a contraindication for transplantation of this tissue.

Question 10: Answers

1 – b
No HLA match is needed for liver, heart or heart/lung transplantation.

2 – f
The cornea is avascular and can be removed up to 24 h after circulatory arrest.

3 – f
The avascularity of the cornea allows this to be possible.

Index

Abdominal aortic aneurysm, 151, 152
Abduction paradox, 119, 120
Achalasia, 189, 190
Acid-base balance, 27, 28
Actinomycosis, 197, 198
Addison's disease, 169, 170
Air embolism, 71, 72
Algodystrophy, 59, 60
Amputations
  foot diabetes and, 137, 138
  knee, 137, 138
  Symes, 137, 138
Anaemia, 31, 32
Anal fissure
  adult, 199, 200
  child, 171, 172
Anatomical snuffbox, 145, 146
Aneurysm
  abdominal aortic, 151, 152
  Berry, 143, 144, 196
  Charcot–Bouchard, 196
  false, 143, 144
  mycotic, 143, 144
  thoracic aortic, 151, 152
Angiography (lower limb), 139, 140
Ankle brachial pressure index (APBI),
  140
Annular pancreas, 172
Antibiotics, indications for use, 9, 10
APC gene, 103, 104
Appendicitis
  child and, 173, 174
  cystic fibrosis and, 35, 36
ARDS, 26, 35
Arterial blood gas, 27, 28
Artery
  facial, 154
  inferior epigastric, 21, 22
  ovarian, 212
  popliteal, 135, 136
  testicular, 212
  uterine, 211, 212
Ascending cholangitis
  presentation, 195, 196
  treatment, 202
Austin–Moore hemi-arthroplasty, 124

Barclay formula, 65, 66
Base of skull fracture, 51, 52
Beck's triad, 48
Biopsy, 13, 14
Bone biochemistry, 121, 122

Bone cysts, 131, 132
Bone tumours, 131, 132
Brachial plexus lesions and anatomy, 129,
  130
  Horner's syndrome and, 130
Branchial cyst, 163, 164
Breast lumps, 99, 100
Brush cytology, 13, 14
Bulbar palsy, 189, 190
Burns
  Barclay formula, 65, 66
  rule of nines, 66

Calcium and bone disease, 121, 122
Captopril, renal artery stenosis and, 5, 6
Carbimazole, side-effects, 43, 44
Carcinoma,
  bladder
    haematuria and, 205, 206
    staging, grading and treatment, 217,
      218
  breast
    TNM Staging, 101, 102
    treatment, 101, 102
  colon
    liver and, 91, 92
    resection margins, 91, 92
    symptoms, 199, 200
  laryngeal, 157, 158
  lung
    hypercalcaemia and, 107, 108
    recurrent laryngeal nerve palsy and,
      157, 158
  oesophageal, 189, 190
  prostate, 221, 222
  renal cell, 205, 206
  thyroid, 105, 106
    FNAC and, 14
Cardiac tamponade, 47, 48, 69, 70
Caroticocavernous fistula, 52
Carotid body tumour, 163, 164
Cervical rib, 81, 82
Chemotherapy, 95, 96
Chordee, 176
Claudication, ischaemic, 135, 136, 139,
  140
Clear cell carcinoma, see Renal cell
  carcinoma
Cloquet's node, 180
Clostridium difficile, Rule of fives, 10
Clostridium tetani, 7, 8
Clotting, 33, 34

Coarctation of the aorta, 81, 82
Codman's triangle, 132
Colostomy, 185, 186–187
Compartment syndrome, 59, 60
Congenital dislocation of the hip (CDH), 125, 126
Constipation in the child, 171, 172
Cornea, transplantation of, 223, 224
Cruciate ligament injury, 127, 128
Cryptosporidium, 43, 44
Cushing's disease/syndrome, 169, 170
CVP line, complications, 71, 72
Cystic fibrosis, 35, 36, 171, 172
Cystic hygroma, 13, 164

De Quervain's tenosynovitis, 113, 114
Deep venous thrombosis (DVT), 135, 136
Developmental dysplasia of the hip, 125, 126
Diabetic foot, 137, 138
Diabetic ketoacidosis, 27, 28
Diaphragm, 75, 76
Digastric, 153, 154
Disc prolapse, 195, 196
Disinfection, 15, 16
Disseminated intravascular coagulopathy, 33, 34
Diverticular disease, 199, 200
Dressings, 25, 26
'Drop Arm' sign, 119, 120
Duct ectasia, 99, 100
Duodenal ulcer, causes of, 169, 170
Dynamic hip screw, 123, 124

Ectopic pregnancy, 191, 192
Elemental diet, 29, 30
Epididymitis, 213, 214
Epiglottitis, 157, 158
Epispadias, 175, 176
Epistaxis, 167, 168
Erb–Duchenne palsy, 129, 130
ERCP, 201, 202
Ewing's sarcoma, 131, 132
External fixation of fractures, indications, 117, 118
Extradural haematoma, 51, 52

Felty's syndrome, 147, 148
Femoral fracture, see Fractures
Femoral triangle, 141, 142
Fibro-adenoma (breast), 99, 100
Finkelstein's test, 113, 114
Fissure-in-ano, 199, 200
FNAC, 14
Foreign body, swallowed, 161, 162

Fournier's gangrene, 7, 8
Fracture
    Barton's, 113, 114
    base of skull, 51, 52
    Bennett's, 113, 114
    Colles, 113, 114
    complications of, 59, 60
    external fixation and, 117, 118
    fixation of, 57, 58
    Hangman's, 61, 62
    Jefferson, 61, 62
    Le Fort, 51, 52
    malunion, 59, 60
    neck of femur, 123, 124
    non-union, 59, 60
    open, 117, 118
    scaphoid, 113, 114
    Smith's, 113, 114
    supracondylar, 113, 114

Gallstones, treatment of, 201, 202
Garden's fracture classification, 124
Gastric erosions, 193, 194
Glasgow Coma Score, 53, 54
Glomerular filtration rate, 207, 208
Grawitz tumour, see Renal cell carcinoma

Haematuria, 205, 206
Haemophilia, 33, 34
Hartmann's procedure, 185, 186
Head injury, 51, 52
Hemi-arthroplasty, Austin–Moore, 124
Hepatitis B, 193, 194, 195, 196
Hernia
    femoral, 179, 180
    inguinal, 179, 180
    obturator, 179, 180
    umbilical/para-umbilical, 179, 180
High dependency unit, allocation of beds, 85, 86
Hilton's White Line, 200
Hip injuries, 123, 124, 125, 126
Hirschsprung's disease, 171, 172
Horner's syndrome, 130
Human immunodeficiency virus (HIV), 43, 44
Hydatid of Morgagni, 213, 214
Hydrocoele, 175, 176
Hypercalcaemia, 121, 122, 170
Hyperkalaemia, 83, 84
Hyperparathyroidism
    calcium and, 121, 122
    paraneoplastic syndrome and, 108
Hypokalaemia, 83, 84
Hypophosphataemia, 83, 84
Hypospadias, 175, 176

Ileostomy, 185, 186
Imperforate anus, 171, 172
Incisions, abdominal, 181–184
Intensive care unit, allocation of beds, 85, 86
Intersphincteric groove, *see* Hilton's White Line
Intravenous urogram, contraindications, 5
Intussusception, 173, 174
Ischaemic bowel, 191, 192
Ischaemic limb, 139, 140

Jejunostomy, 29, 30

Killian's dehiscence, 190
Klumpke's palsy, 129, 130
Knee injuries, 127, 128
Kussmaul's sign, 48

Ladd's bands, 171, 172
Laparoscopic surgery, 21, 22
  contraindications, 202
Le Fort fractures, 51, 52
Leriche's syndrome, 135, 136
Leuco-erythroblastic change, 31, 32
Little's area, 168
Local anaesthetics, 11, 12
Lump in the neck, 163, 164
Lump in the right iliac fossa, 197, 198
Lung function tests, 77, 78

Malaena, 200
Malignant melanoma, 97, 98
Mallory–Weiss tear, 193, 194
Meconium ileus, 171, 172
Meniscus damage, lateral and medial, 127, 128
Mesenteric adenitis, 173, 174
Multiple endocrine neoplasia (MEN), 169, 170

Nasal packing, 168
Necrotising fasciitis, 7, 8
Nephroblastoma, 173, 174
Nerve, anatomy and palsies of
  axillary, 55, 56
  common peroneal, 39, 40, 115, 116
  deep peroneal, 115, 116
  external laryngeal, 39, 40
  femoral, 180
  hypoglossal, 153, 154
  medial and lateral plantar, 115, 116
  obturator, 115, 116
  phrenic, 61, 62
  radial, 55, 56, 145, 146
  recurrent laryngeal, 39, 40, 157, 158
  saphenous, 115, 116, 141, 142
  sciatic, 115, 116, 141, 142
  spinal accessory, 39, 40
  sural, 115, 116, 141, 142
  tibial, 115, 116
  ulnar, 55, 56
NSAID, 109, 110, 193, 194
  asthma and, 5, 6
Nutrition, 29, 30

Oncogenes, 103, 104
Ortner's syndrome, 162
Osteosarcoma, 131, 132

p53, 103, 104
Paget's disease, 132
  biochemistry, 121, 122
Papilloma (nipple), 99, 100
Paraneoplastic syndromes, 108
Percutaneous endoscopic gastrostomy (PEG), 29, 30
Perthe's disease, 125, 126
Pharyngeal pouch, 163, 164, 189, 190
Phlegmasia alba caerula, 135, 136
Phlegmasia alba dolens, 135, 136
Piriform fossa, 161, 162
Pleura, innervation of, 87, 88
Pleural effusion, 7, 78
Pneumocystis carinii pneumonia (PCP), 43, 44
Polycystic kidneys, 195, 196
Porphyria, 206
Portal hypertension, 193, 194
Portosystemic anastomosis, 193, 194
Pott's disease, 198
Pre-operative investigations, 3
Processus vaginalis, 176
Psoas abscess, 197, 198
Pulmonary embolism, 35, 36
Pulmonary oedema, 77, 78
Pyrexia, postoperative causes, 37, 38

Quadrilateral space, 145, 146

Red urine, causes of, 206
Renal artery stenosis, 5, 6
Renal colic
  analgesia and, 41, 42
  symptoms, 191, 192
  treatment, 209, 210
Renal physiology, 207, 208, 219, 220
Resection margins
  colon carcinoma, 91, 92
  skin tumours, 14
Rhabdomyolosis, 83, 84
Riedel's lobe, 195, 196

Rotator cuff injury, 119, 120

Salivary glands, 159, 160
Saturday night palsy, 146
Schistosomiasis, 205, 206
Shock
    bradycardia and, 73, 74
    classification of hypovolaemic shock,
        49, 50
    classification of, 73, 74
    spinal shock, 61, 62
Shoulder dislocation, 119, 120
    axillary nerve palsy and, 55, 56
Sjögren's syndrome, 160
Slipped upper femoral epiphysis (SUFE),
    125, 126
Spleen
    anatomy, 48
    rupture, 47, 48
Splenomegaly, causes of, 147, 148
Sterilisation, 15, 16
Steroids, 109, 110
Stomas, 185, 186, 187
Stones
    renal, 41, 42, 191, 192, 209, 210
    salivary gland, 159, 160
Stridor, 157, 158
Subarachnoid haemorrhage, 195, 196
Subclavian steal syndrome, 81, 82
Subdural haematoma, 51, 52
Subglottic stenosis, 77, 78
Sudek's atrophy, 59, 60
Supraspinatus tendonitis, 119, 120
Sutures, 17, 18
SVC obstruction, 69, 70
Swallowed foreign body, 161, 162

T4, structures found at, 87, 88
Takayasu's ateritis, 81, 82
Tendon anatomy and injury of the foot,
    63, 64
Testicular descent, 175, 176
Testicular tumours, 213, 214

Tetanus, 7, 8
Thoracic aortic aneurysm, 151, 152
Thoracic duct, 87, 88
Thyroidectomy, complications of, 165,
    166
Total parenteral nutrition (TPN), 29, 30
Transient synovitis of the hip, 125, 126
Transplantation, 223, 224
Trethowan's sign, 126
Trigeminal neuralgia, 41, 42
Trigone, 215, 216
T-tube, 201, 202
Tumour markers, 93, 94

Ulcers
    arterial, 149, 150
    Marjolin's, 149, 150
    neuropathic, 149, 150
    trophic, 149, 150
    venous, 149, 150
Ulnar paradox, 56
Umbilical ligaments, 215, 216
Urinary retention (disc prolapse), 196,
    197
Urinary tract infection, 7, 8

Varices (oesophageal), 193, 194
VATER syndrome, 172
Vein
    azygos, 87, 88
    facial, 153, 154
    hemi-azygos, 87, 88
    ovarian, 212
    testicular, 211, 212
Verumontanum, 215, 216
Volkmann's ischaemic contracture, 60
Vomiting, drug treatment of, 109, 110

Wound infection
    classification, 19, 20
    microbiology, 7, 8

Zollinger–Ellinson syndrome, 170

Notes

Notes

Notes

Notes

Notes